Rage-Free
Kids

—⁓⊰∞⊱⁓—

Rage-Free Kids

Homeopathic Medicine
for Defiant, Aggressive,
and Violent Children

Judyth Reichenberg-Ullman, N.D., M.S.W.

Robert Ullman, N.D.

PRIMA PUBLISHING

This book is intended for educational purposes only. It is not intended to diagnose, treat, or give medical advice for a specific condition, or to in any way replace the services of a qualified medical practitioner.

The cases in this book are true stories from the authors' clinical practice. The names of patients have been changed to protect confidentiality. Any names matching or resembling those of real people are coincidental and unintentional.

PRIMA HEALTH and colophon are trademarks of Prima Communications, Inc.

Library of Congress Cataloging-in-Publication Data

Reichenberg-Ullman, Judyth.
    Rage-free kids : homeopathic medicine for defiant, aggressive, and violent children / Judyth Reichenberg-Ullman and Robert Ullman.
    p. cm.
    Includes index.
    ISBN 0-7615-2027-9
    1. Violence in children—Prevention. 2. Aggressiveness (Psychology) in children—Prevention. 3. Conduct disorders in children—Alternative treatment. 4. Homeopathy. I. Ullman, Robert. II. Title.
    RJ506.V56 R45 1999
    618.92'89—dc21   99-16191
                                                                CIP

99 00 01 02 03 04 05 HH 10 9 8 7 6 5 4 3 2 1
Printed in the United States of America

How to Order
Single copies may be ordered from Prima Publishing, P.O. Box 1260BK, Rocklin, CA 95677; telephone (915) 632-4400. Quantity discounts are also available. On your letterhead, include information concerning the intended use of the books and the number of copies you wish to purchase.

Visit us online at www.primahealth.com

*To parents everywhere who are trying
to give their children a healthy, loving start.
And to kids everywhere, who deep down are doing
their best to grow up into healthy adults
despite a not always ideal environment.*

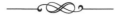

Contents

PART THREE
**True Stories from Our Clinical Practice:
Homeopathic Successes with Defiant,
Aggressive, and Violent Kids**

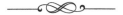

Foreword

West Paducah, Kentucky; Jonesboro, Arkansas; Spring-field, Oregon; Littleton, Colorado. Kids are killing kids in schools across the nation. What drives children to commit such violent, unthinkable acts of murderous rage? The specter of this question haunts the public consciousness of America and the private thoughts of parents who send their children to school each day.

Psychiatrists, psychologists, mental health counselors, public policy advocates, and elected officials argue that easy access to firearms, video and TV violence, parental neglect, poor mental health, and a decline in civility and morals are the primary causes of the unthinkable: children who end up as cold-blooded, calculating murderers. Kids killing kids—this tragic, late-twentieth century American phenomenon is a complex problem that requires complex solutions.

While good public policy can begin to stem the tide of the broader underpinnings of our toxic culture of violence, what hope do parents of aggressive and violent children have for healing their children and leading normal lives? These "rage-aholic" children can suffer from any number of traumas including developmental disorders, central nervous system injuries, family violence and abuse, or parents who may have abused drugs or alcohol. They may be diagnosed by psychiatrists and other physicians as suffering from attention deficit hyperactivity disorder (ADHD), oppositional defiant disorder (ODD), or conduct disorder (CD).

Children carrying these diagnoses manifest their distress differently. Despite the diversity of behavioral presentations, the conventional approach reduces the problem down to a set of single diagnoses typically treated with a limited number of drugs. Practitioners of conventional medicine use stimulant, antidepressant, anticonvulsant, anti-anxiety, anti-psychotic, and a few other drugs to treat aggressive and antisocial behavior in hopes that it will diminish or disappear, often without uncovering the underlying cause of the problem.

Since there is no single medication recommended for the treatment of aggressive behavior, multiple medications have been used clinically to target childhood aggression. This means that if your child has been diagnosed with ADHD, ODD, or CD, he or she may receive one or more potentially toxic drugs with the possibility of severe side effects and drug interactions.

Before you consider using medications to treat you aggressive child, please read this book! The authors, Drs. Judyth Reichenberg-Ullman and Robert Ullman, present a safe and effective alternative to the conventional approach for treating oppostional, aggressive, and defiant children. The Ullmans share their experience in treating over 1,500 children with behavioral and learning problems with homeopathy, often with dramatic success. Homeopathy has been safely and effectively utilized in countries throughout the world for over 200 years. The homeopathic approach treats each patient individually and promotes healing and balance by stimulating the unique adaptive mechanisms within each person. The outcome of the homeopathic course of treatment can improve the function of patients diagnosed with ADHD, ODD, or CD, to the point where prescription drugs are often no longer necessary.

The case studies in this book speak for themselves. Evidence is also accumulating from clinical research studies to support the claims of homeopathy. However, more work needs to be done in this area and the evidence presented by these two pioneers in the field of homeopathy will surely promote increased discussion about the benefits of homeopathic medicine in treating defiant, aggressive, and violent children.

Many conventional doctors remain skeptical about the claims of homeopathy. If you are a parent who needs help with a child similar to those presented in this book, make your own judgments about the safety and effectiveness of homeopathy based on the experience of the Ullmans. *Rage-Free Kids* is a must read for any parent who is facing the difficult decision of whether or not to medicate his or her aggressive or violent child.

Bruce Gryniewski, BS, MA, Ph.D.
Executive Director
The Ceasefire Foundation of Washington

Acknowledgments

We thank the many children whom we have had the opportunity to treat and their parents for trusting us to do so. Our gratitude to Samuel Hahnemann, for having the brilliance and foresight to develop the science and art of homeopathy, and to all the homeopathic masters who have taught us what we know. Special appreciation to Julia McDonald, our acquisitions editor at Prima, Andrew Vallas, project editor, and Kelley Lacey, publicity coordinator, all of whom have been extremely helpful and good-natured. And finally, to Bruce Gryniewski of Washington Ceasefire, for sharing our excitement about this book and for writing the compelling foreword.

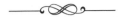

Introduction

We are on the brink of a new millennium. The technological advances that we have made over the past century, and even the past decade, are mind-boggling. One would think that, as we advance as a human race, we would also make tremendous strides in learning to live together in peace—that we could master the art of cooperative co-existence in families, communities, and nations; ensure safety and protection for our children; and mend our differences and move beyond them to create a shared vision of a happy and healthy future for all of us. But this is not yet the case. Despite all of the hurdles we have overcome as a global community, we have not learned to eradicate violence. In fact, in many ways the world seems a more dangerous place than it was in our parents' or grandparents' generations.

In our personal search for peace and harmony, we chose to live in a safe, quiet, and beautiful small town just north of Seattle. It is a place where folks can walk around any time of the day or night and feel relatively assured that no harm will come to them. Imagine our surprise when we read the following report in our local newspaper:

The threat of losing Nintendo apparently proved too much for a twelve-year-old Edmonds boy who was arrested Tuesday after he tried to choke his mother for taking away the controllers to his video game, police said. . . . She had gotten a report from his teacher that he'd failed to do his homework for several days and had been misbehaving in class. When she confronted him, he denied he had any homework, flew into a rage, and attacked her, she reported. A similar incident occurred in Edmonds less than a year ago when a mother tried to take away her son's Sony Play Station. The boy became angry and allegedly tried to strangle her.[1]

One could assume these two episodes are isolated events. But no, even in Seattle where people joke that drivers are just too darned polite for words, our youths are at risk. According to the 1996 *State of Washington's Children* report:

- Twenty-one percent of the state's 1.4 million children will report having been physically abused by age twelve.
- Nearly half of all high school students say they would have no problem obtaining a handgun. By ninth grade, 10 percent say they will be smoking regularly.
- By age 18, half of the kids say they will have access to drugs such as cocaine and LSD.
- Domestic violence arrests, Child Protective Services referrals, arrests for violent offenses by adolescents, and homicide and gun-related deaths in teenagers have doubled, and sometimes tripled, over the past ten years.[2]

The subject of violence in children is currently so much in the public consciousness that vital information is surfacing faster than we can write this book. We would be remiss, however, if we did not mention the excellent article in the latest issue of *Mothering* by Peggy O'Mara, publisher, editor, and a woman we respect tremendously for her pioneering work in the field of parenting. Her editorial cites the January 1999 revised policy of the American Academy of Pediatrics (AAP), following two years of analysis of the subject of children and violence, warns: "Violence has become increasingly prominent in the United States, which has the highest youth homicide and suicide rates among the 26 wealthiest nations in the world and one of the highest rates of homicide worldwide." Despite the fact, as we mention in this book, that the incidence of murders in this country has declined since 1994, violence and violent injuries among children have not. The AAP offers such far-reaching recommendations to pediatricians not only to assess and screen their juvenile patients for such factors as substance abuse, history of mental illness, and family and media factors predisposing to violence, but also suggests advocacy efforts on the part of the physicians on the children's behalf.[3]

Violence is running rampant in our culture and around the world. Aggressive behavior, conduct problems, and antisocial behaviors are far too common among children and adolescents.[4] Rarely a day goes by when newspapers and news reports are not filled with reports of murders, rapes, road rage, ethnic cleansing, and war. "Between 1977 and 1986, the killing of a parent was an almost daily event in the United States."[5] Many of us read in shock about the young man who befriended his well-liked and highly respected high school English teacher and then killed him to steal his bank card. The student and his accomplice stabbed him to force him to divulge his automated teller machine number, then shot him in the head, after which they allegedly withdrew $800 from his account.[6]

Or consider the fifteen-year-old high school student from Springfield, Oregon, charged with four counts of aggravated murder in the 1998 slayings of his parents and two classmates whom he gunned down in his high school cafeteria. This boy, voted by classmates as "Most Likely to Start World War III," was not a gang member or the product of violent peer influences. In fact, his parents were both teachers, widely known for their devotion to kids. They knew their son was in trouble and were sincerely seeking help. Yet their son, who boasted to friends about killing his cat and blowing up a cow, and who built bombs from recipes downloaded from the Internet, was more and more out of control. The day before the murders, the young man was suspended from school when a stolen .32-caliber pistol was found in his locker. Taken to police headquarters and charged with possession of a stolen gun on school grounds, he was released to his parents. That night he shot them dead, then spent the night in the woods. The following morning he strode into his school lunchroom and opened fire.[7]

What could possibly lead a child to contemplate, much less carry out, such acts of violence? Where do the seeds of unconscionable behavior take root? Myriam Miedzian, author of *Boys Will Be Boys: Breaking the Link between Masculinity and Violence*, points out that "over the past decade, arrests of fifteen-year-old boys on murder charges have increased by more than 200 percent, and arrests of boys twelve and under were up 100 percent." (Although incidences are down since 1994).

Not only do many high-risk children go untreated, they see more than 10,000 TV murders by the age of 18, including endless scenes of people shot down, blown up, and burned alive. They develop shooting skills in video games and listen to music lyrics that denigrate women and extol violence. They spend more time being "entertained" than with their parents or in school. No parent can hope to protect his or her children entirely from this onslaught of cultural violence combined with easily available guns.[8]

Everyone is aware of the problem of the senseless violence that surrounds us. We believe homeopathy offers a solution that is largely unknown to the general public. You may be asking yourselves, "So what is homeopathic medicine, and what does it have to do with reducing violence?" Although many of you may be new to homeopathy, you are probably familiar with the term *alternative medicine,* of which homeopathy is a branch. You may have sought out some form of alternative or complementary treatment yourself, or know someone who has. Those using natural medicine are no longer a minority. As a matter of fact, in 1997, 83 million Americans (more than 40 percent of the adult population) sought out alternative medical practitioners. They made more visits to these health professionals (629 million) than to primary care physicians (386 million), at the cost of more than $27 billion.[9] According to a 1993 study in the *Journal of the American Medical Association,* the majority of alternative medicine users appear to be seeking out health care alternatives because they find them to be more congruent with their own values, beliefs, and philosophical orientations toward health and life.[10]

Homeopathic medicine is a particular form of alternative medicine unique to itself. Prior to becoming licensed naturopathic physicians specializing in homeopathy for the past fifteen years, we worked extensively in the field of mental health, and promised to ourselves to find a gentler and more effective answer for mental and emotional problems than conventional psychiatric medications.

Long before entering naturopathic medical school and prior to receiving my master's in psychiatric social work, I, Judyth, had a couple of significant experiences working with at-risk juveniles and adolescents. From 1971 to 1972, I was fortunate to work as a Vista volunteer helping to prepare for college some Upward Bound students in El Paso, Texas. These kids were the firsts in their families to enjoy the possibility of attending college, and, therefore, of dramatically expanding their economic horizons. In 1973 I had my first contact with kids in the juvenile justice system as a supervisor at the King County Juvenile Detention Center in Seattle. I was given the responsibility of supervising half a dozen girls placed there temporarily for a variety of offenses and handed a key to make sure they didn't escape. What I remember most about these girls is that they were simply kids, who, for one reason or another, had gotten off to a really rough start in life, often with little or no guidance.

One of our first experiences in treating an oppositional child was in 1992. Ben, a five-year-old child from Redmond, Washington, had a freckle-covered face and a mischievous grin. "Ben's got warts on his left foot," his discouraged mother told us. "They're just starting to hurt. He grinds his teeth so loudly at night that he wakes us up. He also has incessant tongue lapping. In fact, he does it so often that it creates scabs under his lips. But most of all, Ben is just plain disobedient. We simply can't get him to listen no matter what we try." And no one could say Ben's conscientious parents hadn't tried. In fact, they had tried every parenting method they came across—with little success.

"Ben is a balker. If we say, 'No, you can't,' he loses it. Becomes hysterical. First the crying, then screaming and throwing things. There is no getting through to him. He's downright defiant. Ben pushes and hits whenever he chooses, but if someone does it back to him, he's outraged and yells 'It's not fair!' Going out in public with Ben is humiliating. The public slugging matches are so bad that I'm afraid I'll be accused of child abuse. 'I'm not afraid of you!' Ben challenges at the top of his lungs. 'You're a mean, bad mommy.'

"He's awful with animals. We have to remind him ten times a day to leave our cats and dog alone. His moods can go from black to white in a matter of seconds. It's as if something snaps inside of him. Sometimes he'll get a scowl of his face and shriek, 'Don't touch me!' At other times he can be sympathetic, or he can laugh if another child gets hurt. Ben is fixated on violence—aliens, weapons, movies—and he's constantly asking me, 'Why do the characters want to chop people up?'

"A take-charge type of kid, Ben likes to tell the other kids what to do. Another thing that irritates us about Ben is his endless dawdling. It takes him forty-five minutes just to get dressed in the morning! He stops and starts and asks questions until he drives us crazy. This kid could play 'Guess what, Mom!' for hours on end."

Ben's appetite was enormous. He could eat a full meal, then, less than an hour later, complain, "I'm hungry to death." He had a constant habit of picking his nose; complained of growing pains, gas, and restless sleep; and had suffered from an ear infection after a DPT shot at the age of eighteen months. Ben was also overly sensitive to noise.

Some features of Ben were perfectly typical of five-year-old boys. But other aspects were extreme. The defiance, aggression, moodiness, and absolute disregard for his parents' authority were disturbing. His excessive appetite and nose picking were also out of proportion. We gave Ben a single dose of *Cina* (wormseed) and waited to see his response. Six weeks later his mom reported that the warts on the soles of his feet were completely gone. The lip licking and teeth grinding were considerably less frequent, and his behavior was much improved. "Now he's your normal, average kid," his mother reported. "No more slugging matches or temper tantrums, and Ben is much less defiant. He doesn't accuse me of being a bad mommy anymore. The fixation on violence has diminished, and the growing pains are gone, as is the gas. Ben no longer complains when I touch him. He's still quite noise-sensitive."

Two months later Ben's mother gave another progress report. "He's doing terrific. As perfect as a boy can be. No more warts. Better attitude. Not as rebellious or defiant. His sensitivity to noise is even gone. Even a chain saw didn't bother him." Ben needed four doses of the *Cina* over a year and eight months.

This case made quite an impression on Ben's parents and teachers and on us. We realized that if homeopathy could help this child, who would no doubt be diagnosed with oppositional-defiant disorder, it could hopefully help many others. We have found that to be true. As a result of the overwhelming popularity of our book, *Ritalin-Free Kids,* we have had the opportunity to treat over 1,500 kids with behavioral, emotional, and learning problems. Our practice is outpatient. We do not work with incarcerated or institutionalized youths, although we do occasionally treat children who are on the fringe of the criminal justice system. Most of the kids that we treat for problems of anger and violence are still at the stage of either attention deficit/hyperactivity disorder (ADHD) or oppositional-defiant disorder (ODD), although the minority have moved into the sphere of conduct disorder (CD). We are convinced that homeopathic practitioners can have the most dramatic effect when they treat these children early, which seems to be the consensus among those working with at-risk youths in a conventional setting as well.

We offer our experience in treating these children with homeopathic medicine in hopes that many more children's lives can be turned around for the better. We have spoken with many a devastated and desperate parent. We have felt the chills go up our spines when we hear the stories of kids who lash out with rage at those around them, tormenting animals or people without remorse, and threatening to harm or kill others. The more of these children and adolescents who can be helped with homeopathy or other therapies in their most tender years, the safer, healthier, and happier we can all be.

Rage-Free
Kids

PART ONE

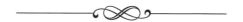

Wrestling with Rage

1

Violent Kids in a Violent World
The Sobering Statistics

"A somber President Clinton said last night that he was 'profoundly shocked and saddened' by the school shooting in Colorado, and he expressed the hope that the country would, somehow, find ways to prevent future bloodshed. 'We don't know yet all the hows or whys of this tragedy,' Clinton said. 'Perhaps we may never fully understand it . . . . The [Littleton] community is an open wound right now.' The president, with face flushed and eyes downcast, went on to express that Littleton is a wonderful place and that if such violence could occur there, it could happen anywhere."[1]

Yet another shocking school shootout. This time, fourteen students and one teacher at Columbine High School near Littleton, Colorado, lay dead, and over twenty others were hospitalized, most of them shot in the chest, back, head, and legs. One girl was wounded nine times. Some hid under tables or in closets, others in ceiling vents, for up to five hours. The lucky ones were able to run for their lives. "We're talking about a war zone," commented one of the parents of an unharmed senior. "It's like walking through a minefield," commented the local sheriff, in reference to a bomb that exploded at Columbine six hours after the shootout terminated with the suicides of the young murderers following their killing rampage.[2]

Heart-wrenching to the families of students who died or were injured, and shocking to those in the local community as well as the world community, this is yet another in a series of violent murders of and by children and adolescents. This nightmare occurred the day we were finishing the manuscript of *Rage-Free Kids*, as if the stories and statistics already gathered for this book were not already convincing of the need for action. "When," we are asking ourselves, "will the killing and violence end?" What can we do to turn around this tragic and senseless trend?

How Safe Are Our Kids?

Most parents would agree that the most essential ingredients of a healthy childhood are love, nurturing, and protection from danger—loving your children and keeping them safe. That is no longer such an easy task. How heartbreaking it is to read the story of a parent who sacrificed to move her family from a drug- and crime-infested neighborhood to a more protected one, only to have her child killed by an errant bullet that went sailing through their living room window. Or to read about kidnappings of youngsters from their backyards or even the sanctuary of their homes, like the case with Polly Klaas, the young girl abducted from her own bedroom whose brutal murder gave rise to a nationwide movement to protect children.

"Disorders of behavior are by far the most common reasons for referral to child psychiatrists, accounting for up to two-thirds of all referrals."[3] From October 1, 1997, to May 21, 1998, even before the Columbine murders, fourteen students were killed and forty-five injured and two teachers killed in eight separate incidents of school violence across the United States.[4] Children are both the victims and perpetrators of crime. The FBI reports that three times as many juvenile homicide victims are killed by adults as by other youths. In 3 percent of murders in this country, both murderer and victim are under eighteen.[5]

Even if parents are lucky enough to protect their children from actual violence, they now have to face the seemingly insurmountable problem of virtual or video violence.

> Imagine your child rumbling into Raccoon City, which is lined with all-night diners, gas stations, and dives, on his Harley-Davidson. Surrounded by policemen firing rounds of bullets. Then bodies slump to the floor twitching and hemorrhaging. Sound far-fetched? Think again. Welcome to "Resident Evil 2," the bestselling sequel to a version of which gamers snapped up more than 500,000 copies for their home computers, and more than two million for video viewing.[6]

It is no longer necessary for your kids to leave the comfort of your home to experience images of death, dismemberment and murder or implied rape. They're the staple of an industry that knows the appetites of the adolescent boys and young men who make up the majority of gamers. Recent advances in 3-D hardware, which can make characters lifelike, have spurred developers to pack titles with even more jarring action.

The mere thought scares some parents almost to death, and leaves them struggling with a contemporary conundrum: how to monitor the games their kids love, the ones that studies suggest may also make them more aggressive, or at least more tolerant of brutality.[7]

A Generation of Children at Risk

According to a 1996 report in our home state of Washington, the following are the sorry statistics about kids in the 1990s:

- At birth: Seventeen percent of newborns are born to mothers who smoked during pregnancy, and 17 percent of newborns are born without appropriate prenatal care.
- By age 10: Forty-four percent of children are not reading at a basic level of comprehension.
- By age 12: Fifteen percent of children personally know adults who deal drugs; 21 percent have been physically abused or mistreated by an adult; 44 percent say it would be "easy" to obtain cigarettes.
- By age 14: Fifteen percent of children carry a weapon for self-defense; 20 percent have thought about attempting suicide; 74 percent say they would have no problem obtaining alcohol.
- By age 16: Four percent are carrying a gun to school; 46 percent say it would be easy to obtain a handgun; 18 percent have been sexually abused.
- By age 18: Thirty-one percent have left home for more than a night because they were depressed or upset; 43 percent know adults who deal drugs; 69 percent say they could skip school without their parents knowing.

Violence Among Children
Is a Problem Worldwide

Aggression and violence among children are serious concerns not only in the United States but throughout the world. We recently visited New Zealand, a beautiful and friendly country at the end of the world. We were told before our trip that New Zealand was much like the United States twenty to thirty years ago, especially in the rural areas, in terms of its lack of complexity and its safety. While visiting the North Island, an article in the Rotorua *Daily Post* attracted our attention. Disciplinary action had been taken against a sixth-grade student after he shot a fellow student in the back with a BB gun at school. He would likely face expulsion. The incident was the first of its type at the school. School principal Bebe Roughton commented, "It was totally unacceptable and a very serious act. The school takes a very hard line against anything which provides a danger to other students. . . . It's not the sort of thing you expect to happen at any school."[9] We fear that this may be a foreshadowing of events to come as New Zealand and other countries "modernize" and "catch up" with the United States.

In Britain 40 percent of seven- and eight-year-olds with conduct disorder become repeat juvenile offenders as teenagers, and over 90 percent of repeat juvenile offenders had conduct disorder as younger children. By the time they grow into adults, their pattern of violence, dishonesty, drunk driving, and unemployment is fixed.[10] "Health service resources [in Britain] spent on children with conduct disorder are considerable: 30 percent of child consultations with general practitioners are for behaviour problems, and 45 percent of community child referrals are for behaviour disturbances—with an even higher level at schools for children with special needs and in clinics for children with developmental delay, where challenging behaviour is a common problem."[11]

Stephen Scott, child and adolescent psychiatrist in London, estimates that aggressive behavior in children (conduct disorder) occurs in nearly 10 percent of children in an urban population and that 90 percent of repeat delinquent offenders have had conduct disorder at age seven. These children are often depressed and fail at school and with friends. As adolescents, their risk of developing an aggressive lifestyle is high as long as they have easy access to an atmosphere of violence. Parenting programs, reports Scott, can be effective in reducing antisocial behavior in children under the age of ten, but adolescents are much more difficult to treat. Despite poor behavior, when the family is supportive, the likelihood of positive change is much greater. Take the case of Winston Churchill, whose school report at age nine described his conduct as "exceedingly bad" but who went on to become a brilliant statesman.[12]

In India where, traditionally, children do not dare contradict or disobey their parents, defiance and disobedience are growing concerns. But consider the following example:

> There's a "Home Alone" cuteness and calm about the face of ten-year-old Rohan Ahuja, but, with the suddenness of a mountain lion, those very delicate features are transformed into a snarl. He hurls abuses and hits out at anything or anyone around him: parents, teachers, classmates at his public school in Delhi. This child sleeps with shards of glass under his pillow and a knife under his mattress. The story goes that he despises his father because he used to beat Rohan's mother. The mother's decision to move out and to remarry only

reinforced this hatred and insecurity. His two wishes: to be a lawyer when he grows up so that he can send his father to jail and to join the underworld so that he can shoot him dead.

Rohan's anger may sound extreme. But he is, increasingly, not alone. . . . Never before has the aggression been so up-front and widespread as it is in the 90s, nor the threshold for tolerance so low. Psychologists and teachers are anxious about the visible increase in the number of acts of violence by children today, whether it is directed at others or toward themselves . . . at any age. Like two-and-a-half-year-old Ramani Krishnan, who kicked the TV set when the electricity went off. Or five-year-old Gaurav Kapoor, who throws tantrums when his mother takes him shopping, kicks and bites her, and threatens to shoot her when she doesn't buy him what he wants. Or Prashant Reddy, a strapping, 14-year-old six-footer who beat up his grandmother, teacher, and the school librarian. A growing number of cases of "social conduct disorder," as psychologists describe aggression, are being referred to therapists by schools. "There is a discernible change in the past five years. I see much lower frustration tolerance in children," says family therapist Bindu Prasad, who counsels schoolchildren in Delhi.[13]

From Acting Out to Murder and Rape

Indicators of future violence in children often begin very early, even as toddlers. There are certain personality traits such as exaggerated selfishness, unwillingness to share or cooperate with other children, frequent and violent temper tantrums, and extreme disobedience and defiance. Next comes a type of dominance and competitiveness that is way out of proportion, intolerance of rules and authority, and maliciousness toward others. The child may have a total disregard for consequences. This pattern can lead to a diagnosis of conduct disorder and, later, juvenile delinquency, which is on the rise.

For example, Rodney Wingate, a custodian of twenty years in the Chesapeake schools in Indian River, Virginia, was not surprised by an occasional broken window. But finding 101 broken windows one night and an additional 66 the next was not only shocking but expensive, costing the school about $6,000. Norfolk, Virginia, schools lost over $107,000 in the 1997-1998 school year to vandals and thieves, topping the annual average of $50,000 to $75,000. School vandalism has no season and no limit. The Virginia Beach school system has responded by instituting a comprehensive prevention program that includes school security managers and guards, nighttime police patrols, alarms, video surveillance cameras everywhere but the restrooms, and classes in teaching kids to think responsibly.[14] All of these measures are a time-consuming and costly solution to an unfortunate problem.

Vandalism is bad enough, but the child-initiated crimes have progressed much further to the unthinkable: murder and rape. Perhaps the most shocking feature of such crimes is the seemingly total lack of conscience or remorse. Take the following example that occurred within half an hour of our home: Two boys, aged twelve and thirteen, were accused of setting fire to Abdirizak Ahmed as he slept on a bus shelter bench in Seattle. The victim, who suffered severe burns over 15 percent of his upper body, still does not have full use of his arms and will need skin graft surgery. Both boys were charged with first-degree assault; however, the attorney for the thirteen-year-old boy, who was diagnosed with attention deficit disorder and oppositional-defiant disorder, argued that his client was incapable of forming intent to cause serious bodily harm.[15]

Or consider this equally disturbing case: "Maddie Clifton knew her 14-year-old neighbor as a playmate and friend. Now Joshua Earl Patrick Phillips sits behind bars, charged with killing the 8-year-old girl and hiding her under his water bed." Alerted by the boy's mother, police found Maddie's body, which had been stabbed at least nine times and struck in the head, apparently with a knife and baseball bat. Joshua confessed and was charged with murder.[16]

Ronald Stephens, executive director of the National School Safety Center, reported that the Jonesboro, Arkansas, murders brought to 201 the number of fatal school shootings since his group began counting in 1992.

> After years of rising violence by juveniles, the recent trend has been a sharp drop in such crime. Juvenile homicide arrests fell 30 percent—from 3,102 to 2,172—between 1994 and 1996, according to Justice Department reports. Nevertheless, crimes such as Jonesboro should be a continuing wake-up call for every school to put together and develop strategies to make school safer.[17]

Appalling though murders by and of children may be, even more unfathomable is rape committed by children. According to Bob Benjamin, a spokesman for the Cook County prosecutor in Chicago, "Around the country, people are finding younger and younger perpetrators of capital crimes. . . . More and more young children seem to be committing sexual assault." Department of Justice figures show a fairly steady increase in rape arrests for children under twelve, from 222 in 1980 (under 1 percent of the total) to 553 in 1996 (nearly 2 percent of all rape arrests). In April 1998, for instance, three boys aged seven, eight, and eleven were arrested in Dallas in the sexual assault of a three-year-old girl who was clubbed with a brick, stripped naked, and left, bleeding, in a creek bed.[18]

Our goal is to make such violent acts by children and adults a rare exception rather than what seems, frighteningly, to be a daily occurrence.

2

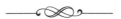

What Makes Kids Aggressive?
The Causes of Rebellious
and Violent Behavior

In our clinical experience, the tendency toward violence and aggression in a child can be evident, or at least probable, even prior to the time a child begins school and enters the social fabric of our culture. Parents of aggressive children often report to us that they first noticed these behaviors in their children's toddlerhoods or infancies. Because we have found that the roots of violence can often be traced back through the family, our habit is to inquire about the state of the mother and father during and prior to pregnancy. Some of the children and adults who are the most enraged are those whose mothers were physically, verbally, or sexually abused during the pregnancy or at the time of conception. Frequently the mother will report to us, "His anger is just like his father's." In many cases, by the time we first see the child the birth parents are no longer together. They may never have actually lived together. Yet there seems to be some thread that ties together the nature of the parent(s) and the child in some inextricable way. And this anger does not even necessarily need to have been translated into action. We have seen cases where violent thoughts held by the parents were somehow passed on to the child either in utero or after the birth. On occasion, the violence in the child can be triggered by a very difficult, painful, and violent labor and birth experience.

Experts confirm our observation that indicators of problem behavior in children are noticeable early on.

> Potential symptoms can be detected as early as infancy—children who can't bond, can't attach to adults and aren't making appropriate developmental gains, says Mary Sarno, mental health program administrator at the Department of Social and Health Services, and cochair of Washington State's SBD [seriously behaviorally disturbed] task force. Early intervention, according to Sarno, can be the key.
>
> "The earlier you can catch a child's problems, the easier it will be to correct it," she says. . . . Hill Walker, an education professor at the University of Oregon and co-director of the Institute on Violent and Destructive Behavior, agrees that studies looking at early intervention corroborate Sarno's conclusion: The earlier the intervention, the larger and more long-lasting the results.[1]

Although it is far too early to confidently diagnose a child with oppositional disorder in the womb, at birth, or even as a toddler, experts agree that by the time a child enters the first or second grade, aggressive tendencies are often obvious. Dorothy Otnow Lewis, M.D., in her review of the research regarding adolescent conduct and antisocial disorder, concludes that aggressive behaviors at the age of eight are good predictors of aggression during adolescence. "Twenty-seven percent of eight- and ten-year-olds who, according to teachers and peers, demonstrated behavior problems, went on to exhibit delinquent behaviors as adolescents. In contrast, fewer than 1 percent of nontroublesome 8- and 10-year-olds later became delinquents."[2]

Are There Such Things as Violent Genes?

The nature versus nurture question arises again. Are children born mean? Do they imitate the behavior that they observe in others? Or are there other factors causing aggression? "For most of this century, disruptive childhood behavioral disorders were assumed to be learned behaviors due largely to environmental factors including poor parenting. However, family, twin, and adoption studies, and the success of medications affecting dopamine, serotonin and norepinephrine metabolism, have suggested an important role for biological and genetic factors."[3] Numerous studies have shown that Tourette's syndrome, ADHD, and drug and alcohol abuse, all of which can potentially result in violent behavior in children, share a number of common genes.[4] However, no single gene has been linked to violence.

The question of whether the like-parent-like-child scenario is due to inherited genes or mimicking of parental behavior is answered to some degree by studies of adopted children who shared common genes with both parents but did not have the opportunity to observe or model their actions.

Associations have been found repeatedly between both childhood disruptive behavioral disorders and adult sociopathy in parents and similar disorders in their offspring. Furthermore, separate genetic and environmental influences—and perhaps a synergistic interaction—have been demonstrated many times for these same disorders. This assertion is supported by an extensive literature consisting of both adoption and twin studies.[5]

Adoption studies of children separated from biological parents at birth tend to show more antisocial behavior occurring in the offspring when a biological parents also has antisocial behavior. In a Stockholm adoption study of 862 men born out of wedlock and adopted to nonrelatives at an early age, there was nearly two times the risk of criminal behavior if either biological parent had a history of criminality.[6]

If violence were a simple matter of inheritance, then perhaps gene splicing would be the ultimate solution. But we have seen a number of aggressive children whose biological parents were calm and mellow, with not an angry gene in sight. There must be more to it than just genes.

Mental Illness and Physiological Imbalance

The American Psychiatric Association estimates that twelve million children have suffered from mental illness, but most don't receive the help they need. "Diagnosing mental illness in children can be difficult because, according to Dr. Michael Witkovsky, assistant professor of psychiatry and pediatrics at the University of Wisconsin–Madison, the symptoms of any single disease can be different from child to child."[7]

Ten psychiatric diagnoses are commonly associated with aggressive behavior in children and adolescents: attention deficit/hyperactivity disorder, conduct disorder, psychotic disorders, traumatic brain injury, seizure disorder, mental retardation, pervasive developmental disorder, depression, bipolar disorder, and post-traumatic stress disorder.[8] We would add to the list sexual abuse, oppositional-defiant disorder, dissociative identity disorder (formerly called multiple personality disorder), panic and other anxiety disorders, borderline personality disorder, antisocial personality disorder, and autism.

According to one study, "Ninety-three percent of the youth in the mental health system who had a diagnosis of conduct disorder had juvenile justice system involvement, yet it was interesting how many youth in both systems had other types of primary psychiatric diagnoses (80 percent)." Those with conduct disorder totaled 21 percent; ADHD 5 percent; adjustment disorder, 12 percent; anxiety disorder, 1 percent; depression/bipolar disorder, 23 percent; developmental disorder, 2 percent; oppositional disorder, 17 percent; personality disorder, 2 percent; psychosis, 3 percent; and posttraumatic stress disorder, 15 percent.[9] What distinguished children with police referrals from other children in the mental health system was a clear set of characteristics—including substance abuse, history of physical abuse, and parental criminal involvement.[10]

The nature and degree of aggression in these individuals varies widely depending on the individual. We may be talking about disruptive classroom behavior in kids with attention deficit disorder as compared to intentional maliciousness in conduct disorder.

Lashing out with anger is a common, impulsive response among children with developmental disorders, as well as manic episodes of bipolar disorder. Among children and adolescents diagnosed with schizophrenia, violence, even murder, can occur, especially when they follow the misguided instructions and messages of their hallucinations and delusions.

"Major mental illness becomes easier to diagnose as children progress in their development at adolescence."[11] Then begins the often agonizing trial and error process of finding the right medicine(s) and the right dosages. It is essential that we understand the causes, manifestations, and likely course of psychiatric problems in children so that they can receive prompt and appropriate treatment within the mental health arena, hopefully before they end up in the criminal justice system.

In addition to mental illnesses, other physiological conditions can cause violent behavior in children and adolescents. They include head injuries, seizures, brain tumors or lesions, psychoactive substance intoxication and withdrawal, and premenstrual dysphoric disorder.[12] In the case of accidents, injuries, and illnesses that affect the functioning of the central nervous system, a carefully taken medical history will elicit a history of recurrent, severe headaches or episodes of dizziness and blackouts (not resulting from the use of alcohol or drugs).[13] Some correlation has been found between behavioral problems in teens and higher levels of androstenedione, testosterone, and disturbed serotonin function.[14] These physiological triggers of aggression are more likely to go unrecognized or to be diagnosed only after other causes are eliminated.

All in the Family

The environment in which children attempt to thrive has a tremendous impact on their attitudes and behaviors. Since family members are enmeshed in so many different ways, it is difficult to sort out just which traits are of genetic origin and which have a more sociological basis. "Families of delinquent children and adolescents are generally found to be unsupportive and unable to cope with transitions and stress, as well as to place less emphasis on such aspects of personal growth as independence, achievement, and cultural and ethical interests than families of nondelinquent children." More mother-child conflict and parental discord, beyond divorce or separation, is correlated with children diagnosed with conduct disorder. Antisocial personality disorder, criminal behavior, and alcoholism, especially in the father, are the more consistently reported family factors that increase the child's risk for conduct disorder. The mothers of these children frequently suffer from antisocial personality disorder, somatization disorder, or alcohol abuse.[15]

Low socioeconomic status is a predictor not only of conduct disorder but of delinquency.[16] The primary risk factors for juvenile justice system involvement among youth in the mental health system include ethnicity (overrepresentation by African Americans), history of physical abuse, parental incarceration, and drug/alcohol involvement.[17]

More specific factors implicated in a child's environment relative to violence later in his or her life are birth position (with middle children having a greater risk compared with first-born, youngest, or only children), social class (which includes other factors such as family stresses, poverty, and family size), harsh or inconsistent disciplinary techniques (which may include a high incidence of child neglect or abuse), and quality of education.[18]

Abuse Breeds Aggression

Children respond to abuse in diverse ways: some retreat within, others strike out, and still others dissociate partially or entirely from the experience. One of the most extreme acts of violence, engendered to a significant degree by severe abuse, is parricide (the killing of a parent). This is not as rare an event as you might think. "Between 1977 and 1986, more than 300 parents were killed each year. In this group, 15 percent of mothers, 25 percent of fathers, 30 percent of stepmothers, and 34 percent of stepfathers were killed by sons and daughters under eighteen."[19] The professional literature suggests that parricide is committed by three types of individuals: (1) the severely abused child who is pushed beyond his or her limits, (2) the severely mentally ill child, and (3) the dangerously antisocial child.[20]

Many of the children we have treated for aggressive behavior have themselves been victims of some form of violence or abuse. Although violence in families probably represents a greater detriment than all genetic disorders combined, it has still not achieved anywhere near the scientific recognition. Differentiating the causes and effects of domestic violence from related issues, such as inadequate parenting, homelessness, poverty, substance abuse, and neighborhood and school violence, is a tough call for researchers. This is especially true because more than one form of violence or abuse can occur at the same time in the same family, and members of the family can be either victims or perpetrators or both, depending on the circumstances. Violent families tend to produce violent kids. "Exposure to violence in the home is linked to juvenile crime. Conduct disorder and antisocial behaviour, even at the age of seven, are powerful predictors of violent behaviour toward partners in adolescence and early adult life."[21]

Abuse in any form, not only that inflicted on the child directly, can have a lasting and detrimental impact. A Punjab University study of 200 children between the age of six and eight revealed that as many as 80 percent of antagonistic children admitted their parents were either aggressive or violent toward each other.[22] "If Daddy can abuse Mommy," the child learns, "I can treat my wife [or anyone else, for that matter] aggressively when I grow up."

Another form of abuse that can be devastating for children, and can inspire them to express violence themselves is peer abuse. In our earlier book, *Ritalin-Free Kids*, we give the example of a young Japanese boy who was so terribly tormented by relentless bullying that he committed suicide.[23] Researchers have found that children who emerged as aggressive after being bullied by peers four to five years earlier were more likely to have experienced a punitive, hostile, and abusive family environment than those children who turned out to be more passive.[24]

It is not only physical and emotional abuse but also sexual abuse that provokes violent behavior. "The histories of severely behaviorally disturbed aggressive children reveal, again and again, a pattern of physical and/or sexual abuse. Unfortunately, most of this abuse goes unrecognized and unreported and hence rarely elicits protection from the state."[25] An estimated 114,000 cases of sexual abuse were substantiated by child welfare authorities in the United States in 1994, approximately 44 to 73 percent of whom were likely to receive some form of counseling or psychotherapy in the aftermath.[26]

Some of these children will respond to sexual abuse in kind by becoming perpetrators of sexual or physical abuse themselves. Several years ago we received a chilling request from a prison inmate for homeopathic treatment. He recounted, with candor and in grammar-school English, how he had been made to do sexual things by his stepfather against his will. The upshot of his abuse was his commission five years earlier of an act so violent that he has been incarcerated. He refused to reveal the exact nature of his crime, saying only that he had done something really bad. We explained that we would need the authorization of prison officials to provide any treatment, and did not receive any further communication from the young man.

Substance Abuse

Another significant factor that may cause, or more often overlap with, aggressive behavior in kids is alcohol and drug abuse. The greatest risk for developing a substance abuse disorder occurs between ages fifteen and nineteen.[27] At least 5 percent of adolescents qualify for the diagnosis of an alcohol use disorder.[28] Both increased aggressivity and conduct disorder are associated with a greater amount of alcohol consumption by underage adolescents.[29] Conduct disorder is only one of the psychiatric problems implicated in adolescents with alcohol dependency. In addition to a greater incidence of disruptive behavior disorders, these children also have a greater risk of mood and anxiety disorder. Children who are antisocial and/or aggressive are more likely to later develop alcohol and other substance abuse problems.[30]

We have found that children with alcoholic parents are much more likely to turn to alcohol and drugs to solve their own problems. Another complicating factor in a number of the adopted children we treat is fetal alcohol syndrome, which frequently does not show up in its full-blown form until the child is school age and, to an even greater degree, during adolescence. Aggressiveness is only one of many problems of children exposed to excessive amounts of alcohol during pregnancy.

It is critical that these adolescents receive the treatment that they need. Too often they end up in the criminal justice system prior to being identified as substance abusers. The longer the problem continues undiagnosed and untreated, the less likely help will be found.

Thrill Kill: Does the Media Model Violence?

It is impossible to open up a newspaper, be subjected to movie previews, or sit through an hour of television (commercials included) without being bombarded by many visual and sound bites of action-packed violence. Are kids able to selectively tune out these images afterward, or do they make a memorable and lasting impression on their psyches?

Where do child and adolescent murderers, like the youngster from Oregon mentioned earlier, get the idea to kill?

Kip Kinkel was found guilty of murdering two students at Thurston High School in Springfield, Oregon, and wounding twenty-five others, only hours after he killed his parents. Apparently *South Park,* Kip's favorite television show, could always make him laugh. In fact, he even tuned in to the program in the company of his dead parents. In *South Park,* Kenny, a fourth-grader, is killed week after week, only to reappear in each new episode.

Larry Bentz, principal at Thurston, warned that we need to stop denying that the level of violence in the media desensitizes kids to violence. "I'm not talking about just films—I'm talking about video games, the newspapers and the news. You see these kids who live in front of those video games and they're blowing characters away, and they come back to life as soon as you turn the button back on. How can that not desensitize kids to violence?" Springfield school superintendent Jamon Kent added, "I know that our kids come to us already seeing something like 13,000 killings on television."

Video games may actually train children to commit violence, in the opinion of Dave Grossman, a retired U.S. Army lieutenant colonel and author of the book *On Killing*. Grossman, who teaches psychology at Arkansas State University in Jonesboro, was among the first counselors to arrive at Westside Middle School after the shootings there in March, 1997. "We've taught our children to kill and we've taught them to like it." Go to a theater, he suggests, "sit through a horror film, and watch the audience. You will see children too young to be there, and they will laugh at the gore, because they are conditioned to find it pleasurable."

School murders in Kentucky and Washington do seem to have at least one common pop-culture connection: Stephen King's *Rage*. In the book, a boy takes his class hostage and murders his teacher, just as fourteen-year-old Barry Loukatis reenacted when he donned a long, black gunfighter's coat and killed two students and a teacher in Moses Lake, Washington. Loukatis's mother had also shared with him her violent fantasies of kidnapping her husband and his lover at gunpoint, tying them up, and making them watch as she killed herself.[31]

According to Jeffrey B. Pine, former attorney general of Rhode Island in 1992:

Kids are literally bombarded with messages in the media, be it the six o'clock news, tabloid television, video games, or movies; they're saturated with violence. When you add to these influences such other factors as substance abuse, the availability of handguns, and the breakdown in the confidence of certain community institutions, it's really not any wonder that by the time a child is 6 or 7, he or she has been saturated with violence and not with values.[32]

Despite the fact that the impact of the effects of television violence on children and adolescents was first brought to light as an issue in the 1950s, it is only recently that it has been recognized widely as a public health concern. Numerous studies document that mass media violence contributes significantly to aggressive behavior, fear, and desensitization of violence.[33] More than 1,000 studies substantiate a correlation between media violence and aggressive behavior in children.[34]

Leonard Eron, a psychologist at the Institute for Social Research in Michigan, and his colleagues, have been studying over 800 people beginning in 1980 when the individuals were eight years old. Over the decades, they found that, compared with boys who watched fairly mild TV shows, boys who watched violent programs were more likely to be aggressive as adults and to bearrested for drunken driving and felonies.[35] One of the most compelling pieces of research was the National Television Violence Study (1995 and 1996), commissioned by the National Cable Television Association.[36] The researchers arrived at the following conclusions:

- Handguns were featured in 25 percent of all violent scenes.
- Violence usually goes unpunished on American television.
- Seventy-three percent of perpetrators failed to experience negative consequences for their actions.
- Humor often accompanies violent scenes.
- Only 4 percent of programs actually condemned the use of violence.
- Only 15 percent of violent programs carried any kind of advisory or content code.
- Public broadcasting stations carried the least amount of violence and cable channels the most (85 percent).

The study found 75 percent of music videos to contain sexually suggestive images and 56 percent to contain violence, mostly directed against women. "Many music themes are worrisome and include sadism, masochism, incest, devaluation of women, graphic violence, the occult, drugs, alcohol and suicide as an alternative or solution."[37]

Even if exposure to media violence doesn't lead so far as instilling aggression in youngsters, it can still have damaging effects. Professor Sudhish Pauchauri, in a study on TV and society in Delhi, found that children, as passive consumers, are mesmerized by ad jingles and must have what they want at any cost. "Many of the ads aimed at children show that muscle and bluster get you what you want: If you want Babul bubble gum, the quickest way is to brandish a gun. If you want another kid's toffee, just snatch it."[38]

Jeanne B. Funk, one of the few child psychologists to study the effects of game violence on children's behavior, found that children who spent the most time playing violent games have lower self-esteem. They see themselves as less popular, less skilled academically, and less athletic.[39]

Is the Boob Tube Any Less Violent Than Video Games, Videos, and Movies?

If, as a parent, you console yourself with the fact that your child is much more likely to spend his free time plopped in front of the television than going to a movie, you are right. The researchers of the national TV violence study concluded that, "Although movies are far more graphic than is television, the average child watches only one or two movies per week, compared with 23 to 27 hours of television." Lest you feel too complacent about entrusting your child to the so-called boob tube, many studies have attested to the relationship between exposure to television violence and an increased likelihood of aggressive behavior.[40] The Lion & Lamb Project, a long-range study of 875 children, concluded that watching violent television programs in the children's early years resulted in later aggression, including violent criminal offenses, child abuse, and spousal abuse.[41]

A visiting scholar at Harvard University's Graduate School of Education founded Action for Children's Television (ACT) in 1968. The 10,000-member non-profit organization worked to encourage program diversity and eliminate commercial abuses in children's television.

In large part, commercial television has abdicated its responsibility, its education role. And instead, it concentrates on its ability to amuse. Many adults are understandably frustrated and angry with the commercial television fare that showcases meaningless violence, raunchy rock rhymes and sexual innuendo. They are deeply concerned about television's connection to murder and mayhem in our neighborhoods and schools. They want the government to ban violent adult movies and to take away G.I. Joe's guns and Ninja Turtles' swords.[43]

The methods suggested to foster change are cited in the sidebar on page 30.[44]

Bombarded by the Boob Tube

The following eye-opening statistics were compiled by TV-Free America (printed in "Students Look Elsewhere During TV Turnoff Week" by Wendy McKellips in the *South Whidbey Record*).[42]

- Ninety-eight percent of American households own at least one television, which is turned on an average of seven hours, twelve minutes per day.
- The average child spends 1,680 minutes each week watching TV, compared to 38.5 minutes a week engaging in meaningful conversation with her parents.
- Only one parent in twelve requires his or her child to finish homework before watching TV.
- The average child has viewed 8,000 TV murders by the time he has finished elementary school and 200,000 violent acts by age eighteen.

Parents Fight Back against Violence

Many parents have felt relatively helpless in the face of their children's fascination with media violence. Media murders seem to be everywhere. In 1997, a fourteen-year-old freshman at Heath High School in Paducah, Kentucky, opened fire on a group of students just as their prayer group was breaking up. Three students were killed, and the boy, who pleaded mentally ill to murder and other charges, was sentenced to life in prison. The families of the three victims have recently sued twenty-five entertainment companies for $130 million. They alleged that violent computer games, Internet pornography, and *Basketball Diaries,* a Leonardo DiCaprio movie, contributed to the vicious attack. The film includes a dream sequence in which a student guns down a teacher and his classmates. Included in the group being sued are Nintendo, Sega, and Sony.[45]

A Multifaceted Problem with a Multifaceted Solution

In 1994, Senator John H. Chafee of Rhode Island discussed the correlation between violent crime and the availability of handguns. Although he admitted that violent crime was on the downswing from 1993 to 1994, he expressed concern that criminals were increasingly likely to be armed with guns and that offenses committed with pistols and revolvers rose from 9.2 percent of crimes in 1979 to 12.7 percent in 1992.[46] Senator Chafee specifically addressed the subject of teen violence in the form of suicide:

Combating TV Violence

- Hold local stations accountable for providing quality children's programming by reminding them that failure to provide educational choices for children will result in the station losing its license.
- Seek out the good programs.
- Encourage the television industry to ban ads for violent movies during children's program time.
- Increase funding for public broadcasting.
- Fund day care programs.

The Committee on Communications made some additional suggestions in the respected journal *Pediatrics,* in an attempt to prevent adverse impact from the mass media on youngsters:[47]

- Produce more educational, nonviolent programs.
- Creatively depict violent acts being punished.
- Highlight alternatives to the use of violence.
- Watch television with children and discuss the issues that arise.
- Understand the role of television in children's socialization, and the potential risks.
- Take into account a child's developmental level when making viewing decisions.
- Use program advisories and other content information in deciding which programs to let your child watch.

There are 22,500 Americans murdered every year, but more than 25,000 Americans take their own lives every year. And handguns are the leading instrument used, with 12,700 handgun suicides.

Teenagers are particularly susceptible to suicidal impulses, and a gun in the home more than doubles the chances of a teenager successfully committing suicide.[48]

How much of this violence among our teens happens in schools? According to a recent report by the Department of Education, over 6,000 students were expelled in 1996 and 1997 for bringing guns to their schools. A 1995 study by the Centers for Disease Control and Prevention (CDC) indicated 8 percent of all students reported bringing a gun to school in a thirty-day period. One handgun control organization estimates that forty-four incidents of violence in U.S. schools involving firearms were reported in the media from September 1998 through May 1999.[49] Although President Clinton has done much to support the cause of regulating firearms, only fifteen states in the U.S. have child-access-prevention laws requiring gun owners who live in households with minors to lock their guns out of the reach of children.[50]

Regardless of the specific factors that are engendering a climate of childhood and adolescent violence, Jeffrey B. Pine, former Rhode Island attorney general, summed it up aptly:

We all have to recognize that we have a serious problem, and frankly, an entire generation of young Americans is at risk. We also have to accept individual responsibility for this and realize that collectively, we have a stake in our children's future. It's not the other person's problem; it is *our* problem. And each of us in our own way and in our community has to be willing to step up and be part of the solution, whether from education, from law enforcement, from the medical community, from the health care industry, whatever it may be. . . . [51]

3

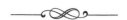

Desperate Parents
Living with a Difficult Child

We receive calls from parents all over the United States as well as from foreign countries requesting our help. They plead to consult with us immediately. "Our situation is urgent," they lament. We can hear the tension in their voices. Some mothers are crying. They use phrases like "We're at the end of our rope" or "You are our last hope." They feel such pressure from the school system, discord in the home, and imminent danger to or from the child that it seems to them a life-or-death situation. And, as is evident from the statistics we cite here, that impression may be justified. Once we interview the parents and child, they often ask that we send the medicine by overnight mail. The feeling is "We can't go on like this for another day." "Your book has given me hope," they confide—hope of escape from the nightmare of living with a difficult and dangerous child.

"I Can't Believe He's My Child"

It is often depressing and shocking for parents to realize they have a violent child. "Where did we go wrong?"

they ask. "Was my child born without a conscience? We tried to instill correct moral values, but he doesn't have any feeling for other people. How did he end up that way?"

We treat one child whose mother operates a kennel. She dare not turn her back for fear that Sam would torment one of the dogs. She adores animals and showers them with love and affection. It is beyond her comprehension that Sam could even consider hurting another living creature. Yet he did until we were able to help him with homeopathy. Even worse for some of these parents is the child's total lack of remorse. It is bad enough, they reason, to harm another creature. But to have no idea that such an act is wrong or to even derive pleasure from seeing another's pain is inconceivable to many parents.

"Who, Me? I Didn't Do Anything"

One of the most aggravating features of angry and aggressive children is their lack of responsibility for their actions. No matter what they have done, regardless of the consequences and whether any person or property has been damaged, there is often no admission of guilt or responsibility. In fact, these kids often claim *they* are the victims. "He did it to me" or "They're always picking on me" or "It's not fair" are excuses that we hear most commonly. This victim stance not only drives everyone else away but is often firmly ingrained into adulthood. The child is always looking for someone else to blame and for some reason to explain away her actions. The reason that ADHD, ODD, and CD are included under the grouping of disruptive behavior disorders is that the child's actions generally cause more of a problem for those around them than for themselves (although this is less often the case with ADHD in which children can feel very bad about their learning deficits and behavioral inappropriateness). It can be very hard to live with a child who blatantly abdicates any responsibility whatsoever for her actions.

"I Can't Trust a Word He Tells Me"

Trust is one of the principal foundations for interpersonal relationships. We need to be able to count on those around us. We care about them and, in turn, want to know that they will in turn be caring and trustworthy. One of the most discouraging features of rebellious and defiant children is their tendency to lie. At the beginning, these lies are a way to keep them from getting into trouble for doing something they know they shouldn't have done: "No, I didn't eat those cookies" or "Yeah, I brushed my teeth"—little fibs that they hope will never be discovered. "After all, they'll never know if I really finished my homework," such a kid thinks.

Next come the bigger lies: "No, I don't know what happened to that twenty dollars that was on your dresser." "Sure, I went to school today." "Yeah, I passed my math exam." Or, a few years later, "No, I'd never touch a cigarette." "We went to Bernie's house after school. His mom was there the whole time."

It's amazing how kids can lie with a straight face. We see twelve-year-old Craig for depression. We've given him several medicines with only a partial response. It was puzzling to us since the medicines should have helped him. We've even asked him directly, without his mother present, "Are you sure you're not doing any drugs?" "Nope," Craig assured. "No drugs." He seemed like a kid you could really believe. We got a call from Craig's mom last week. It turns out that he's been secretly smoking marijuana for over a year.

In extreme cases, children can become pathological liars. We have seen this to be particularly true in children from broken families whose father or both parents were drug or alcohol abusers and lied habitually. Children like this lie so frequently about so many aspects of their daily lives that even *they* don't know what to believe. And their parents lose trust in the children because half of what comes out of their mouths is untrue.

"He's Ruining Our Lives"

Sadly, this is a comment we hear with some frequency. The difficult child does not only cause problems for himself and his parents but for the rest of the family and for those beyond the immediate family. After the parents, next affected are siblings. The challenging child may be provoking, taunting, or even abusing his brothers and sisters, even to the point of creating lasting or permanent psychological scars. Another major concern of parents is that these difficult children may be setting an example or a role model, however negative, for the younger siblings. They may start imitating his fixation on violence, foul language, and rebelliousness toward anyone in authority.

Then come the family pets, who may react to being teased, tormented, or even tortured either by withdrawing or by becoming mean and aggressive themselves. "Tracy just can't understand why our cat won't go anywhere near her" or "We had to give away our bunny because we were afraid Cameron would strangle her."

The neighborhood children can also become the targets of a nasty or aggressive youngster. They may feel intimidated to the point where they are afraid to go out and play with him. It may bring out their own bullying tendencies. Or, if sexual abuse is involved, they may receive profound harm that they are terrified to discuss even with their parents.

Classmates are so affected by a problem child that their parents forbid him from going to their houses or demand that he be expelled from school to prevent harm to their own kids. These children can so completely upset the balance and relative harmony in a family or social system that the parents no longer know how to cope.

"We Never Have a Moment of Peace"

Having a challenging child in the family may seem like way more than a full-time job. Cindy and Kevin Cormier were the wasted parents of their challenging child, Christian. Diagnosed at three with ADHD, Christian was described as having a Jeckyll and Hyde personality. "Just imagine," explained Kevin. "It's a light switch, and you turn it on and you get the bad side; you turn it off and you get the good side. And that's how fast it happens . . . just like that." Mealtimes were agonizing confrontations during which Christian's parents would beg him to sit down and share the family meal. Bedtime was a war of wills and strength lasting up to five hours. Kevin and Cindy avoided taking Christian out in public and rarely had time for their younger son, much less for each other.

The child's explosions erupted several times a day, often deteriorating into a gut-wrenching, all-out battle.

Cindy described the analogy of her son being in the driver's seat with his parents under the wheels. Christian punched, kicked, screamed, and spit for hours on end despite being on medications that were supposed to calm him down. They finally found a doctor who correctly diagnosed him with oppositional-defiant disorder and recommended that they limit their battlegrounds with Christian, pretty much letting him eat and do what he wanted, within limits. Dr. Greene counseled the parents that Christian might need to be on medication for life. Christian's behavior improved, although it leads one to wonder just how he would manage in life if everyone around him didn't do everything his way.[1] It is likely that homeopathic treatment could have helped this child in a more profound way.

Our hearts go out to parents of aggressive and defiant kids. No matter how hard they try to turn around the situation, they often feel they have failed. After this struggle has persisted for a number of years, these parents may reach the point of illness, exhaustion, or divorce. Finally, in cases where every moment of the family's attention and energy revolves around one problem child, especially when danger of physical harm is involved, the parents may decide they can no longer keep the child at home. Sometimes homeopathy can result in a dramatic improvement so that the family can be preserved intact. At other times, for the sake of the family as a whole, the child needs a placement, often temporary, outside of the home.

"I Can't Reason with Her"

Life in a family is composed of an ongoing series of events requiring give-and-take on everyone's part. Because each person's needs may be different, getting along smoothly is a matter of negotiation and compromise. Also essential is respecting the needs of others in the family. This all assumes reasonability on everyone's part or, in the case of children, as much as can be expected for their age.

Some children are downright unreasonable. Parents complain that they don't listen, don't care, and will not cooperate, even with the smallest request or demand. This can turn even the smallest task such as taking a bath or going to bed into a battle. The problem is that the battle never ends. One defiant moment after the next. All day long.

"We're Afraid He'll Hurt Us"

We remember one adolescent whose parents brought him in for a consultation. Jeremy was extremely angry at his rule-setting, policeman father. They had made the appointment with us after he had a physical confrontation with his dad. He had clenched his fist and threatened to punch him, which was the last straw for his firm father. In talking with Jeremy, not only did he not respect his father, but he hated him. Jeremy experienced recurrent violent thoughts about what he would like to do to his father. Rather than sincerely listen to Jeremy's feelings and concerns, his father tightened the clamps by taking away privileges, which served only to fuel his son's hatred. We saw Jeremy only twice, after which his parents sought out other treatment. It would not surprise us, unless the situation significantly changed, if Jeremy would at some point attempt to hurt or kill his father.

We have heard many other stories recounted by parents regarding their children's threatening behavior toward them and others. One twelve-year-old killed small animals, licking the blood off the knife that he used for hunting. He threatened his mother with violence regularly. She brought him to see us out of fear that she might be the next victim. Another child, four years old, tried to smother her newborn brother with a pillow. Still another, at five, shoved his little sister in

"He Is Out of Control"

There are many ways that parents describe kids whom they just can't handle. These are some of the descriptions that we have heard:

- "He goes ballistic."
- "She gets this wild, crazed look in her eye."
- "He goes off on me."
- "No baby-sitter can handle him."
- "The teacher said we either put him on drugs or he's out of school."
- "We cannot take her out in public."
- "I say 'black' and he says 'white.'"
- "If homeopathy doesn't work, we'll have to put him in an institution."

These are kids who refuse to be disciplined. No matter what is asked of them, the answer is "No!" They are often nasty, rude, insulting, selfish, and domineering. Their inner pain and loneliness are masked by outrageously inappropriate and disruptive behavior. We are not just talking about kids who got a rough start in life. They may have been raised in the seemingly ideal, loving home. The conscientious parents may have sought out all kinds of assistance to no avail. In the end, if they have not succeeded, they may feel at a dead end with few remaining options.

the clothes dryer when she made him angry. A lively little girl swung the family's pet bird over her head in a purse, accidentally killing it.

Whether out of benign impulsivity or malicious intention to harm others some children are capable of hurting others severely. Parents are, with good reason, afraid to leave these kids alone with other siblings or family pets. What a terrible and terrifying quandary it is to fear for your own life at the hands of your child.

Too Desperate for Words

Fortunately most of the parents of the children we treat are usually able to get a handle on their own anger, although we know this is by no means universally true. They attend parenting classes, seek family therapy, get all the help they can from the school system, and sometimes seek homeopathic care for themselves as well as their children. The following is a story of parents who felt pushed way beyond their limits.

Angeline and Michael Rogers of Brillion, Wisconsin, pleaded guilty to felony child abuse charges of having kept their seven-year-old daughter in a dog cage when they were unable to control her. Judge Steven Weinke, recognizing that the parents were overwhelmed by the daunting task of caring for five children ranging from one-and-a-half to eleven years of age, sentenced the couple to a year in the county jail with time off or weekly counseling sessions and up to sixty hours of work a week. Before pleading guilty to confining their daughter, the parents were each charged with ten felony counts alleging abuse of four of their children. Prosecutors alleged that the couple had beaten their four older children with a drain pipe and wooden sticks. All five children were subsequently placed in other homes.[2]

Never Give Up Hope

Yes, there sometimes are good reasons to feel desperate. It is an understandable reaction to a difficult situation. But there are a number of options short of going crazy or getting rid of your kid. This book is meant to instill hope and to provide another alternative. Between homeopathy and all of the conventional therapies and interventions, you can hopefully find a solution short of institutionalization or the criminal justice system. Be persistent in your search to find answers for your child and your family. Finding the resources that you need may take considerable effort, but the sooner you are able to find help, the better for all involved.

4

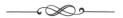

Reasons Behind Rage
What Kids Tell Us and What They Need

To a homeopath, each child or adult is a unique, special human being with particular motivations and feelings leading to subsequent actions. No two violent children are the same. They need to be understood as individuals. This phenomenon of individuality, which is at the heart of homeopathic treatment, has been recognized by some in the mental health profession. "Three 8-year-old boys were brought for psychological help. Their behaviors were very similar, but their actual problems were very different." Tommy, Avi, and Jon were described as unfocused, unable to listen and respond appropriately, underachievers, and socially immature. Now "each of these boys is a well-functioning, high-achieving fifth grader. Treatment approaches were very different for each of them, because their underlying problems were different."[1]

It is only through crawling into the skin, so to speak, or walking in the shoes of that child that we can begin to understand how he feels. Spitting, kicking, screaming, sulking, defying, deceiving, stealing, raping, murdering—to the homeopath these are all actions or expressions. What is most essential in helping the child is to discover what is the feeling that lies beneath or behind the expression. Everyone has such an underlying feeling that often runs as a thread throughout his or her life. By sharing some of the feelings that youngsters have confided in us, we hope to impart the flavor of some of the inner states that motivate a child toward violence. These feelings present, in a sense, the other side of the story. Remember that what is on the inside is not always evident from the outside. In other words, these kids may be shrieking or throwing things at you or threatening to kill you. But underneath the anger is a deeper feeling.

With each of these themes we also share observations of what these kids might need on an emotional level. It goes without saying that, with any of these states, we recommend homeopathic treatment. Homeopathy stands an excellent chance of shifting these states even if they have taken hold on the psyche of the child or adolescent for years.

"Nobody Loves Me"

At the core of many children who lash out with violence is an underlying feeling of loneliness. In terms that adults are more likely to use, they feel unlovable. They realize, although it may not always be apparent, that they are pushing people away. They don't want to do so but don't know how to stop. They may have experienced abandonment by a parent or someone else close to them and have never gotten over it. They feel that they lack support, love, encouragement, and affection, whether or not that is actually true.

These kids need love, pure and simple—in any form, at any time, even if they seem to reject it. The challenge is that they are not always lovable, nor are they necessarily able to communicate that love is what they seek. We recently spoke to Barbara, the mother of Carissa, whom she had adopted at the age of one day. The mother subsequently gave birth to Reanne. She remarked on the drastic difference between the two children. Carissa rejected the affection of her mother, acted in a standoffish and rude manner, and defiantly shouted, "You're not my real mommy so I don't have to do what you say." Barbara's other child was the warm, affectionate little girl that she had hoped Carissa would be. When Barbara returned from a week's vacation in New York, Reanne raced to hug her mom while Carissa ignored Barbara, which she found quite painful.

However, although it appeared that Carissa didn't care, whenever Barbara got ready to leave Carissa's day care after dropping her off, Carissa grabbed onto her legs for dear life and screamed bloody murder for her not to leave. Finally, one day Carissa broke down in sobs and was able to express, at least momentarily, that Barbara really was the mommy that she loved. This is a child who, deprived of the love of her birth mother, desperately wanted the company and nurturing of her new mom but was afraid or unable to ask for what she needed. Carissa has recently begun homeopathic treatment and is already able to more honestly express her feelings and needs.

"Everyone Is Cruel to Me"

Kids can be very mean to each other. They tease, taunt, and call each other cruel names without a second thought. For some kids, these insults roll off like water from a duck's back. But for sensitive children who already feel self-conscious and inadequate, cruel words can be like poison. They may cry or refuse to cry for fear of making matters worse, or they may exhibit somatic symptoms like headaches or stomachaches that prevent them from having to go to school. Worse still, they may internalize the cruelty and begin to believe those terrible things about themselves. Before long they can become victims, responding passively to everything and everyone in their lives.

Sometimes these children need lessons in how to stand up for themselves and fight back. They must be encouraged to ignore what is said. After all, it's easy targets that appeal to most bullies. Kids who can defend themselves or just don't engage in the conflict are no fun to tease. A change of school may be necessary in some cases, but you want to make sure the same situation isn't re-created in the next one.

"I Feel Powerless"

Surprising though it may seem, some of the most malicious, remorseless acts committed out of rage are due to helplessness and a perceived loss of power. Take, for instance, children who have been repeatedly abused. Beaten year after year, unable to escape, their grudge becomes deeper and deeper. They have no way to strike back or get even—until one day they find a gun or some other weapon with which they can feel powerful. All of the rage built up for years explodes. That is when everyone loses.

Empowerment in whatever form is appropriate is likely to help. In the case of physical, verbal, or sexual abuse, the child needs an escape route, a way out. That may be through foster care or the mother standing up to the abusive father. If a sibling is the abuser, the two may need to be separated. In some cases, bedrooms at opposite ends of the house may be sufficient. If the abuse persists, the abuser may need temporary or permanent placement outside the home, whether in foster care or a live-in educational or treatment institution.

"Life Sucks"

These children see only the worst in everything, sometimes with good reason. They may have been dealt a bad hand, gotten off to a bad start in life from which they never recovered. The feeling is that nothing will change, things will only stay as bad or get worse with no ray of hope. Self-esteem is poor, and, in the extreme case, it seems as if there is no reason to live. These kids are depressed.

Anything that makes these children feel good about themselves is helpful: a friend, counselor, hobby, pet. Something that will bring meaning and purpose to their lives is essential to restoring self-esteem and a positive feeling about life.

"I've Been So Hurt"

These are sensitive children who feel deeply hurt, but they may not show it. Their tendency is more to retreat and withdraw. They may be angry inside and often do not reveal the source. It may be hurt from a sibling whom they feel doesn't care, from a boyfriend or girlfriend, a teacher—anyone they perceive to have injured them.

The best course with these children is to love and support them and to provide a safe atmosphere for them to share their feelings when they're ready.

"I Feel Betrayed"

Betrayal is a very intense emotion that often carries with it a quality of life or death about it. It often results from a strong charge that may in turn spur a desire for revenge. Jealousy is often involved, and sometimes lying. It is a feeling of being treated unfairly, of being wronged. These kids harbor bitterness and resentment. Such sentiments, if fueled, can lead to retribution.

These kids need to be heard. This is a good time for active listening—that is, fully hearing them out. Sometimes they just need to vent their anger. If, however, the bitterness runs deep and continues to feed on itself, professional counseling, in addition to homeopathy, may be more helpful.

"Everything Makes Me Mad"

There are children and adolescents who are angry about everything. They express an underlying hypersensitivity and general irritability. Everything anyone else says or does is a cause for antagonism and contradiction. No one else can do anything right besides them. They may be so determined to prove you wrong that it's not even worth playing their game. Touchy, cross, nasty, rude— just mad. But usually they're hurting inside. They don't really want to alienate everyone with their nastiness, but they do, nevertheless.

Often a deeper feeling will emerge if they're willing to talk and you're willing to listen. Otherwise, loving them, being consistent, and setting limits on how much you and your family members are willing to be abused by them are appropriate, as is counseling, if they are willing to talk to anyone about what's really bothering them.

"I Hate Myself"

This is one of the deepest and most disturbing core issues among children. And it can be difficult to elicit because you may only see the superficial anger. These kids believe that they are losers or that they have done something terrible. Extremely demanding of themselves, they are often without friends. This may be the result of rejection or scorn by a loved one, or it can be a deep feeling that arises without any obvious cause. It is particularly disturbing because, especially in the teen years, it can lead to suicidal thoughts or attempts.

Self-loathing is a deep pit and is likely to need the help of a mental health professional experienced in working with depressed children. Give these children as much love as you can, and remind them of all the things you see that are positive and deserving of love even if they can't see the goodness at the time.

"I'm So Afraid"

One of the most common emotions underlying anger is fear. In fact, the more intense the rage, the more intense the terror. Sometimes it is a specific fear, such as being alone or in the dark or being killed. At other time it's more global. These kids may lash out with terrific bursts of rage, biting, scratching, and kicking. But many of them will be terrified inside. The fright often originates from abandonment or perceived abandonment at a very early age.

The best solution for this fear is to make sure these children know they are safe and to make any adjustments in their environments to keep them safe if they are not already.

"I'm Stupid"

This is a refrain we hear very often from aggressive children with ADHD. Because of their problems with paying attention, concentrating, and sitting still, they frequently have difficulty keeping up with the other kids, both academically and socially. Their difficulties are not intentional but may appear to be due to their obliviousness, impulsiveness, and sense of being out of control. This perspective is compounded by what seems like everyone being on their case, especially parents and teachers.

It doesn't do much good to tell these kids how bright they are because they don't believe it. It's best to try to understand what makes them feel this way then, if possible, to directly address their concerns. If it is poor performance in school, get them whatever help they need, including individual educational plans or private tutors or a different classroom teacher or school. If it's low self-esteem, they may need counseling and to find something that they're really good at and love. The worst thing you can do with these kids is to reinforce their already damaging beliefs by criticizing them every time they screw up.

We realize that with very angry kids it is much easier said than done to try to see beneath their rage to the underlying feelings. But we have found that this is much more effective than to just manage their anger without addressing the deeper cause. Remember that, somewhere inside of all these children, they want to be loving, lovable, kind human beings. Try to see them that way.

5

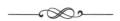

Dedicated Doctors
Using Drastic Drugs
Whatever Works

Psychiatrists, pediatric neurologists, family practitioners, and psychologists are all faced with the problem of
what medications to use to treat oppositional, aggressive, destructive and violent kids. Although a variety of
medications including stimulants, antidepressants, an-
ticonvulsants, and antihypertensive and antipsychotic
medications are all used for these and related conditions, there is no single, effective pharmaceutical solution for children who have oppositional defiant disorder
or conduct disorder, characterized by opposition, behavior problems, moodiness, and aggressive or antisocial behavior. Many times a combination of drugs is
prescribed, each of which is used to address an aspect of
the child's problems in an attempt to provide a partial or
more complete solution.

The main problem with conventional medications
is not that they are ineffective. Most of them do produce
measurable effects on the conditions they are prescribed
for, but at what cost to the child? Side effects can emerge

such as changes in appetite, growth retardation, tics, weight gain or loss, sleep problems, drowsiness, dizziness, blurred vision, headaches and stomachaches, diarrhea, irritability, moodiness, agitation, tardive dyskinesia (antipsychotics), and addiction (benzodiazepines). Parents are understandably concerned about the side effect issue, while desperately searching for a solution for their children's problems.

Parents and doctors, without being aware of or accepting of the benefits of homeopathic medicine, are faced with making a trade-off between the potent main effects and the sometimes limiting or detrimental side effects of conventional medicines. As we review the standard treatments for childhood mood and behavior problems, it will become clear why safe, nontoxic, effective homeopathic treatment can provide a more acceptable solution.

Oppositional and Aggressive Psychiatric Disorders

Mental and emotional disorders in children are an enormous problem for parents, schools, and society.

> The American Psychiatric Association estimates that 12 million children have suffered from mental illness, but most don't receive the help they need. . . .
> "Diagnosing mental illness in children can be difficult. The symptoms of any single disease can be different from child to child," said Dr. Michael Witkovsky, assistant professor of psychiatry and pediatrics at the University of Wisconsin–Madison.[1]

Within the spectrum of childhood mental illness, the disorders involving opposition and aggression make up a large portion of the caseload of mental health practitioners. "Aggressive behavior, conduct problems, and antisocial behaviors encompass one third to one half of all child and adolescent psychiatric clinic referrals."[2]

Children who exhibit oppositional behavior and aggression are given a variety of diagnoses depending on the specific features and symptoms that they exhibit, though the majority of *aggressive* children fall under two diagnostic categories: ADHD and CD. Children who are merely oppositional, but not aggressive or destructive, are classed under ODD. As we have already discussed in chapter 2, children with violent tendencies can be classified under a variety of psychiatric diagnoses and often more than one at a time.[3]

The ADHD Connection

Before we elaborate on which drugs are used for particular diagnoses, it is necessary to clarify the diagnostic catagories of ADHD, ODD, and CD, as well as other conditions that produce violent behavior.

Although ADHD is often found in both oppositional and aggressive children, not all children with ADHD are violent or even oppositional. ADHD has three main components: poor attention, impulsivity, and hyperactivity. These may be present in varying degrees in individual children, and aggression may be an accompanying characteristic or codisorder.

Although aggression is not a specific criterion for diagnosis, there exists a large overlap between attentional deficits/hyperactivity and conduct problems/aggression. Inasmuch as ADHD and conduct disorder (CD) co-occur in 30 percent to 50 percent of cases, it is common to find aggression as a chief clinical complaint in children presenting for psychiatric evaluation with underlying ADHD.[4]

When the distractibility, impulsivity, and hyperactivity of ADHD children are combined with negative, violent, or destructive attitudes or behavior, the child can be completely unmanageable and dangerous to both himself and others. Plus, the frustration often evident in ADHD children can explode into anger, rage, and violence in stressful situations. Episodes may be intermittent or continuous, depending on the severity of the child's mood and behavior disorder.

Nasty and Negative

Oppositional defiant disorder is in the middle of the spectrum, between ADHD and conduct disorder. Dr. Timothy Wilens of Harvard Medical School offers a very good description of children with this disorder:

> While children who have oppositional defiant disorder will not necessarily be depressed, they will appear to have a pretty consistently negative attitude, taking the opposite side against you, teachers or other authority figures, being quick to blame others for their behaviors, frequently swearing, acting like "tough guys" and being annoying to or being annoyed easily by others.[5]

According to Wilens, a large group of these children will grow out of their oppositional behavior, but some of the rest may go on to develop conduct disorder, even while quite young.

Kids Without a Conscience

Children with conduct disorder are often described as "juvenile delinquents" (technically a legal term) or "children without a conscience." These children and adolescents are often cold, callous, cruel, and hurtful. Aggressive and violent, they tend to erupt in outbursts of rage that may or may not be provoked, causing harm and damage to people and property. They lie, steal, get in fights, and break things. With no respect for authority or rules, they go after whatever they desire with no thought of consequences and no sense of responsibility or guilt for their bad deeds.

Psychosis, Seizures, and Developmental Disorders

Other disorders that frequently result in childhood aggression are psychotic, seizure, and developmental disorders. In psychosis, the child may hallucinate, hear voices, have difficulty thinking, and feel disconnected from reality. Paranoid reactions may lead to aggression and violence if the child has a delusion of persecution. She may hear voices telling her to perform a violent or destructive act, or imagine that a harmless person is actually following or attacking her.

Some seizure disorders, particularly temporal lobe epilepsy or complex partial seizures, may mimic psychosis and lead to depersonalization, moodiness, rage, and bizarre, sometimes violent outbursts.[6]

> The relationship between aggressive behavior and epilepsy remains controversial. . . . A positive association between epilepsy and aggression in children has been supported by several studies . . . . However, the association between aggression and seizure disorder diminishes when co-occurring psychosocial and neurologic risk factors are controlled.[7]

Children with developmental disabilities such as mental retardation, autism, and pervasive developmental disorders may become aggressive if stressed. The pervasive developmental disorders (PDD) are a varied group of conditions that share these characteristics: severe and pervasive difficulty with mutual social interaction, verbal and nonverbal communication, or rigid, often repetitive behavior and activities, depending upon the age and level of development of the child. Other features may include mental retardation, seizures, and disruptive behaviors, such as excessive aggression, impulsivity, temper outbursts, and self-injurious behavior (SIB).[8]

All children with developmental disorders are by no means violent, but a significant minority can exhibit extremely oppositional, defiant, and aggressive behavior that can make their management and care a real challenge.

Stressed, Depressed, Moody, and Brain-Injured

Posttraumatic stress disorder (PTSD), bipolar disorder (BD), depression, and traumatic brain injury (TBI) cases account for most of the rest of defiant, aggressive and violent children. Children with PTSD have experienced a significant life trauma, often involving a brush with death or serious injury to himself or the injury or death of someone close to him. This generates an extreme fear, desire to escape, and helplessness. The trauma is so deeply imbedded in the subconscious mind of the child that the painful event is often re-experienced over and over again. Consciously or unconsciously, the child often makes every effort to avoid meeting with such a situation again. The shock of the traumatic event often leads to mistrust, acts of aggression, poor bonding with caregivers, and a sense of isolation in these unfortunate kids.

Children diagnosed with bipolar disorder often exhibit extreme moodiness and may have features of depression and agitation together, unlike adults in whom they are usually well separated. When the two states collide, aggression can be the result. "In children, mania commonly takes the form of an extremely irritable or explosive mood, sometimes psychosis, with poor social functioning that is often devastating to the child and family."[9]

Brain-injured children can have a wide range of deficits and problems, including moodiness and aggression, depending on the part of the brain that is affected.

Traumatic brain injury (TBI) is a prevalent health problem in children and adolescents. Five million children sustain head injuries each year in the United States and 2,000 to 5,000 remain severely handicapped. . . . Aggressiveness, explosive outbursts, and irritability are highly associated with TBI and a major source or stress to families. Aggression is often triggered by trivial stimuli, does not usually involve premeditation, serves no clear goal, is explosive in quality, and intermittent in frequency.[10]

The randomness of the aggression and its unpredictability are major challenges to the family of the child with TBI.

Finally, depressed children may also be irritable, explosive, and aggressive toward others. "Rates of depression among psychiatrically-referred children and adolescents vary between 7 percent [and] 30 percent and become more frequent with advancing age. Irritability and aggression can be a common symptom of depression, especially in males."[11] Depressed children and adolescents, however, are more likely to exhibit self-injurious, even suicidal, behavior than outright aggression. According to a 1996 State of Washington's Children report, by age fourteen 20 percent (of children) have thought about attempting suicide.[12]

Drastic Drugs

The drugs used to treat children for oppositional defiant disorder and conduct disorder are the same drugs used to treat attention problems, psychosis, epilepsy, bipolar disorder, hypertension, depression, and anxiety. These drugs have some effects, particularly on related problems, but:

at present, there is no single medication to recommend for the treatment of aggressive behavior. Multiple medications have been used clinically in a nonspecific fashion to target excessive childhood aggression. Although successful for some, this approach increases risk for ineffective interventions accompanied by side effects.[13]

What psychiatrists and other physicians tend to do is to treat the other conditions surrounding the aggressive and antisocial behavior in the hopes that the unwanted behaviors will also diminish or disappear. The main drugs used for this purpose are the stimulant drugs such as Ritalin (methylphenidate), Dexedrine (dextroamphetamine), and Adderall, which treat the ADHD components; antidepressants, either tricyclics or selective serotonin reuptake inhibitors (SSRIs) such as Imipramine, Prozac (fluoxetine), or Zoloft (sertraline); high doses of strong seizure drugs such as Tegretol (carbamaxine) or Depakote (valproic acid); antihypertensives such as clonidine and Tenex; beta-blockers such as propanolol; anti-anxiety drugs such as Buspar; and potentially addictive benzodiazepines such as Valium, antipsychotic drugs such as Haldol, Mellaril, and Navane, and Lithium, usually used for bipolar disorder. This means that if your child has ADHD, conduct disorder, or oppositional defiant disorder, he may receive one or more potent, potentially toxic drugs, with the possibility of severe side effects and drug interactions.

Significant and Serious Side Effects

Physicians have to be extremely careful with selection of drugs and dosage to avoid creating new problems while trying to cure the presenting disorder. Though the side effects of conventional medicine are more often annoying and rarely life threatening, several of the drugs can have long-term side effects. The stimulant drugs may cause growth retardation in some children and tics (small, repetitive involuntary movements), which usually go away in time but may not disappear in some cases. Tardive dyskinesia, a more serious, permanent side effect caused by long-term use of psychotropic medications such as Thorazine, Haldol, Mellaril, and Stelazine, causes involuntary muscle movements and Parkinson-like symptoms such as a shuffling gait. These drugs are used as a last resort when other drugs are not able to control aggression.

Minor, annoying side effects abound with nearly all psychiatric medications. The amphetamine stimulant drugs—Ritalin, Dexedrine, and Adderall—cause primarily appetite suppression and sleep disturbance. This is not surprising, as Dexedrine (dextroamphetamine) was originally marketed as an appetite suppressant and as a means to combat drowsiness and increase alertness for mental tasks. The stimulants may also cause stomachaches, headaches, irritability, sadness, and a rebound hyperactivity when the dose wears off. Cylert (pemoline), a slightly different kind stimulant, has been known to cause liver problems and needs careful monitoring.

The tricyclic antidepressants can cause "dry mouth, constipation, sedation, headaches, vivid dreams, stomachaches, rash and blurred vision."[14] These drugs should not be stopped suddenly, or vomiting, diarrhea, and stomach cramps may result.

The newer SSRIs have their own set of disturbing side effects. These drugs include Prozac (fluoxetine), Zoloft (sertraline), Paxil (paroxetine), Luvox (fluvoxamine), and Celexa (citalopram). Psychiatrists are the first to admit that SSRIs are not perfect. According to Dr. Timothy Wilens, author of *Straight Talk about Psychiatric Medications for Kids,* "The most common side effects of these medications include: agitation, stomachaches and diarrhea (gastrointestinal symptoms), irritability, behavioral activation, headaches, insomnia, and less commonly, sedation."[15]

Other antidepressants include Wellbutrin (bupropion), Effexor (venlafaxine), Desyrel (trazodone), Serzone (nefazodone), and Remeron (mirtazapine). Wellbutrin has stimulant-like side effects. Effexor can cause nausea, agitation, headaches, stomachaches, and high blood pressure; Desyrel and Serzone can cause confusion, constipation dry mouth, agitation, and sedation.

The MAO inhibitors are an older group of antidepressants including Parnate (tranylcypromine) and Nardil (phenelzine) that are not as often used in children because of the necessity of avoiding tyramine-containing foods such as aged food and cheese, over-the-counter cold medicines, and some recreational drugs including cocaine and ecstasy.[16]

The antianxiety drugs also have side effects and may be addictive. Valium (diazepam), Librium (chlordiazepoxide), Klonopin (clonazepam), Xanax (alprazolam), and Ativan (lorazepam) are benzodiazepines. They are effective in controlling anxiety or panic disorder but possibly addictive with long-term use. A newer drug, Buspar (buspirone), is an antianxiety drug that can also help aggressive behavior in kids with ADHD and pervasive developmental disorders. It has fewer side effects than the benzodiazepines but may be less effective in combating anxiety.

The antihypertensive (blood pressure–lowering) drugs, including Catapres (clonidine), Tenex (guanfacine), and the beta-blockers such as propanolol, are being increasingly used in children for psychiatric purposes, including sleep problems, control of tics, impulsivity, emotional outbursts, and aggression. These drugs dampen the adrenergic part of the nervous system, which helps control these behaviors. Clonidine can cause excess sedation, irritability, and depression. Tenex can result in irritability, sadness, and confusion if the dose is too high. If both drugs are stopped too quickly, the child's blood pressure may rise. The beta-blockers are used to help phobias, aggression, and severe impulsivity. Side effects are mostly gastrointestinal, but depression, hallucinations, and vivid dreams occur in some children. Blood pressure and heart rate may also be affected. Propanolol should not be used in children with asthma or diabetes, nor should it be discontinued suddenly.[17]

Mood-stabilizing drugs include lithium carbonate, the anticonvulsant drugs Tegretol (carbamazine) and Depakote (valproic acid), and the antipsychotic drugs such as Haldol (haloperidol), Mellaril (thioridazine), and Stelazine (trifluoperazine). These drugs are used most often in children and adolescents who have severe mood swings, emotional outbursts, uncontrollable aggression, and, in some cases, psychosis.

Of these drugs, lithium is probably the most benign. It is effective in bipolar disorder and some cases of aggression, and its side effects are relatively minor when dosage is controlled properly, which requires blood-level monitoring. Gastrointestinal symptoms, sleepiness, tremor, memory loss, and kidney problems resulting in excessive urination and thirst are the common side effects.

Depakote and Tegretol, though used to control seizures, also have a stabilizing effect on severe mood swings. Often given in high doses, these drugs may have significant side effects, including gastrointestinal symptoms, blurred vision, dizziness, depression of the immune system, and liver toxicity. Careful monitoring of blood levels is essential.

The numerous antipsychotic drugs are usually re-
served for cases uncontrolled by other medications because of their often severe and sometimes long-lasting
side effects. The reversible side effects are drowsiness,
dizziness, dry mouth, increased appetite, weight gain,
and constipation. More serious symptoms include
Parkinson-like symptoms such as masked face, shuffling
gait, tremor, and the uncontrollable involuntary movements of tardive dyskinesia with long-term use, both of
which may be irreversible.

What Is a Parent to Do?

Reading the list of side effects in the previous section
should give even the most desperate parent pause. It is
not our intention to condemn parents for making the
choice to use conventional medication for their children's serious behavior problems. We honor the efforts of
both parents and physicians to do what is best for the
children under their care. Some children benefit greatly
from conventional medication with few or no side effects, and many side effects are reversible simply by discontinuing the medication.

What if you could achieve the same or even better
results through the use of a safe, nontoxic form of medicine such as homeopathy? Wouldn't it be worth investi-
gating to see whether your child could benefit? Our
experience shows that, in many cases, it is worth trying
a different approach, especially if you are already uncomfortable with the effects, or side effects of pharmaceutical drugs or conventional treatments have been
unsuccessful for your child's behavioral and learning
problems.

PART TWO

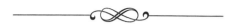

Homeopathy: Safe and Effective Natural Medicine

6

About Homeopathy
What It Is and
Why You Should Know About It

If you are new to homeopathy, you are probably wondering what it is all about and how it can be of help to you and those you love. You may have many questions about this very different, unique form of medicine, and the answers may surprise you.

Homeopathy is an entire system of medicine based on the idea of using very small doses of natural substances to stimulate the body's ability to heal itself. It is based on the principle of "like cures like," also known as the "Law of Similars." Homeopathy is a one-of-a-kind medical approach differing from conventional medicine in both theory and practice (see sidebar on following page).

Homeopathy is not new. In fact, it has been practiced continuously, and in much the same way, for more than two hundred years in many parts of the world, including Europe, North and South America, and India. The theories and practices of conventional medicine have changed hundreds of times during the same period, but the technique of homeopathic prescribing has stably endured the test of time.

What Is Homeopathy?

Homeopathy:

- treats the whole person as a unique individual
- prevents and cures illness rather than merely suppressing symptoms
- is safe and effective for people of all ages including babies, the elderly, and pregnant women
- treats mental and emotional as well as physical symptoms with a single medicine
- promotes a feeling of energy, well-being, and creativity

Homeopathic medicines:

- are almost entirely natural rather than synthetic, derived from mineral, plant, and animal sources
- are used in very small doses and often given very infrequently, the effects of each dose acting for months or years in chronic illness
- do not have the toxic side effects of conventional pharmaceutical drugs

The Discovery of Homeopathy

Homeopathy was created and developed by a brilliant, opinionated, and very dedicated German physician named Samuel Hahnemann (1755–1843), who could best be described as a medical renegade. Hahnemann had his own ideas about health and medicine and was extremely critical of the rather barbaric medical methods of his time, which included bloodletting, leeches, vomiting, and the use of strong purgatives. He was appalled by these drastic measures and hoped to find a gentler, more effective form of healing. As a physician, chemist and medical translator well-versed in both ancient and modern medical thought, he tried to understand the fundamental process by which healing occurs. Making detailed observations of his patients and their illnesses, he developed the theory of healing called the "Law of Similars."

Hahnemann found that any substance in nature capable of making a healthy person sick is able, conversely, to make certain sick people well. Not only are many obviously toxic substances such as arsenic, mercury, insect, spider and snake venoms, and strychnine able to cause poisoning or even death, but these potential killers also can be made into valuable, lifesaving medicines, capable of curing a wide range of ailments. Even ordinary substances that are capable of causing symptoms in healthy people can be made into homeopathic medicines. Homeopathic medicines are drawn from all corners of the world and from every conceivable natural substance. Mineral substances including oyster shell, table salt, and gold; plants such as club moss, comfrey, and windflower; animals, particularly their blood and milk; and insects are all grist for the homeopathic mill. All these substances, poisonous or ordinary, and nearly two thousand more, become potent medicines when properly prepared and used according to the Law of Similars.

The Homeopathic Healing Power of Natural Substances

The key to the homeopathic healing power of natural substances is to understand the particular set of symptoms that each is capable of causing in a healthy person and also curing in a sick person. Each substance has a unique pattern of symptoms, called its *symptom picture*. For example, a bee sting causes certain readily observable symptoms with which nearly everyone is familiar: heat, stinging or burning pain, swelling and redness—the classic signs of inflammation.

By the principle of like cures like, honeybee (*Apis mellifica*) should be a medicine for illnesses with these very symptoms, and so it is. *Apis,* when made into a homeopathic medicine, is used to treat allergic reactions, pink eye (conjunctivitis), arthritis with pain and swelling, and, of course, bee stings.

The picture of a homeopathic medicine is derived from experiments called *provings* conducted on groups of healthy volunteers, as well as by observing what symptoms have been cured in actual clinical practice. In a proving, dilutions of the substance are given repeatedly to each volunteer until the person develops symptoms, which are any alterations in the body, mind, or emotions. Examples of symptoms are a crushing headache in the back of the head, perspiration on the forehead, a desire for oranges, and dreams about running from the police. All of the symptoms from all of the volunteers are collected and compiled to form the picture of the homeopathic medicine. When the medicine is used on patients, all of the symptoms that are cured are also noted, and additions are made to the symptom picture.

Stimulating a Healing Response

Homeopaths use this information to prescribe a single homeopathic medicine that is able to stimulate a healing process that cures or, at least, improves the illness. Homeopathic medicines are prescribed based on all of the symptoms that a person is experiencing at a given time. The whole person is taken into account, not just his or her physical body.

The imbalances in a person's mind and emotions play an equal and sometimes greater role in determining the necessary homeopathic medicine. That is why homeopathy can still treat mental and emotional illness even if the patient is physically healthy. In this book you will see cases where the children have absolutely no physical symptoms, just rage and defiance, and other cases where asthma, allergies, digestive problems, earaches and other childhood illnesses are present. Homeopathy treats the whole person, no matter what is out of balance or causing the behavioral or physical problems.

Treat the Person, Not the Disease

The biggest difference between homeopathy and conventional medicine is the emphasis in homeopathy of treating the person, not the disease entity. Homeopathy attempts to balance and strengthen the individual's own ability to withstand challenges from stress, the environment, and microorganisms. No attempt is made in homeopathy to kill invading organisms; to suppress the body's natural response to disease; or to chemically alter the heart, brain, lungs, liver, kidneys, or other organs and tissues of the body. Instead, the homeopathic medicine provides a template for healing, fostering a healing response and restoring, if possible, the normal condition of body and mind.

Homeopathy views symptoms of disease as an attempt by the defense mechanisms of the body-mind to restore balance and health. Fever, for example, is not the disease itself but a sign that the body is trying to restore balance. To suppress the fever with aspirin or acetominophen, unless it is high enough to be dangerous, is to rob the body of the very tool it needs to defeat the microorganisms. A skin rash or eruption can be an attempt by the body to eliminate waste matter, pus, or other material through the skin. If the rash is suppressed by corticosteroids, the body must seek another means of waste disposal at a deeper level, such as the kidneys, liver, or lungs. This suppression may lead to a more serious illness involving more vital organs, such as asthma, colitis, or kidney disease.

How Homeopathy Works

The fact is no one knows the mechanism by which homeopathic medicines work, only that they do indeed produce results that improve health and well-being. Scientific research into homeopathy has demonstrated statistically significant clinical effectiveness in many health conditions, but *how* the changes happen remains a mystery. A review of 107 research studies in homeopathy was conducted by a team of Dutch medical researchers and published in the prestigious *British Medical Journal* in 1991. The review evaluated the effectiveness of homeopathy reported by studies on health conditions such as respiratory infections, hayfever, rheumatoid arthritis, acute childhood diarrhea, and psychological problems. The authors concluded that of the twenty-two studies that were deemed methodologically acceptable, 80 percent showed positive results for homeopathy.[1]

Various theories have been proposed to account for the results of homeopathic treatment, but none have been accepted as a definitive mechanism. Significant prejudice in the scientific and medical communities and limited access by homeopaths to major research institutions hinder a fair evaluation of the underlying mechanism and effectiveness of homeopathic medicine. For example, work by Dr. Jacques Benveniste on the effect of microdoses of antigen on immune cells known as basophils aroused a storm of controversy several years ago, because it suggested an explanation for the homeopathic effects of microdoses. Beneveniste's results were ridiculed, retracted, and vilified after their publication in the prestigious journal *Nature,* but he was eventually vindicated when his research was replicated and republished in the *Journal of the French Academy of Sciences.*

Conservative members of the scientific and medical communities, except perhaps in parts of Europe and in India, often consider homeopathy to be an archaic hoax at worst and the placebo effect at best. Open-minded scientists and physicians may be more willing to entertain the possibility that homeopathy works, but many are reserving judgment until a precise mechanism of action can be scientifically verified and replicated. Research in homeopathy, mostly clinical in nature, is currently being conducted around the world (see chapter 12). Perhaps when a critical mass of research studies has been achieved, there will be a more general acceptance that the homeopathic phenomenon is indeed real and effective in many cases and for a wide range of illnesses and conditions. Over one hundred studies regarding the clinical effectiveness of homeopathy have not been sufficient to convince skeptics, who continue to insist that there is no scientific validity to homeopathy. This is patently untrue, yet we hear this criticism repeatedly. While we are strong supporters of further homeopathic research, we wonder just how many studies will be enough to convince the critics that homeopathy can and does work. Two hundred? Five hundred? Time will tell. Regardless of how many studies have or have not been completed to date, as you will see from the cases in this book, homeopathy can achieve startlingly positive results in children and adults with behavior problems as well as physical illnesses.

The Single Medicine

People are often surprised when they hear that homeopaths only use one medicine at a time and that one medicine can stimulate the body to heal nearly everything wrong with a person at a given time. Homeopaths have great conviction in a person's ability to heal him- or herself when properly stimulated by the correct homeopathic medicine. This belief is born of the practical experience of witnessing the global healing response brought about by a single homeopathic medication, affecting the whole person: body, mind, and emotions.

Why is only one medicine selected? One medicine has the best chance of matching the patient's symptoms exactly and stimulating the body to heal itself. In chronic illness, most homeopaths find the best results with a single medicine that matches nearly all of the symptoms of the patient. As long as it works, the same medicine is usually prescribed whenever it is needed. If the symptom pattern changes, however, a new medicine is selected that matches the new symptoms. Both medicines are not used at the same time, because each matches a particular set of symptoms. Only the medicine that actually matches the symptom picture at a given time will act to promote healing.

Even so, combinations of homeopathic medicines may work, especially in acute illnesses, when that combination happens to include at least one medicine that closely matches the person's symptoms. However, using the single homeopathic medicine best indicated during an acute illness is likely to produce more dramatic and longer-lasting results and is always recommended for chronic disease.

Microdoses Have Big Effects

Another aspect of homeopathy that is confounding to many people, including the scientific and medical communities, is how small the doses are of homeopathic medicines. Homeopathic medicines are prepared by a process of serial dilution and shaking from an extract of the original substance called a *mother tincture*. For a plant medicine, a mother tincture is prepared by soaking the plant in alcohol for a prescribed period of time. The resultant extract is then diluted according to a particular dilution scale. The most well-known scales are the decimal (X), centesimal (C), and fifty-millesimal (LM) potencies. In X potencies, one drop of extract is added to nine drops of water or alcohol and shaken. For C potencies, one drop is added to 99 drops, and for LM potencies, one drop is added to 50,000 drops of diluent. The most common is the C potency scale. C potencies come most commonly in 6C, 12C, 30C, and 200C and also in 1M, 10M, 50M, and CM potencies. The number indicates how many times the medicine has been diluted: 200C has been diluted two hundred times, 1M has been diluted one thousand times, and 10M has been diluted ten thousand times, still in the C scale of 1:99

drops. The *M* in this case refers to the number of dilutions, not the scale, which can be confusing at first.

The nearly unbelievable part comes when we cal-
culate the actual concentration of the original substance
after the dilution process. After twelve dilutions, or
12C, the concentration is 10^{-24}, exceeding Avogadro's
number (the number of molecules in one mole of a given
solution) and effectively eliminating the possibility that
any molecules of the original substance remain. For example, 12C is a low potency in homeopathy, meaning
not many dilutions. Imagine the concentration at two
hundred, one thousand, or ten thousand dilutions—it is
astronomically small.

A chemist would say nothing remains in such a dilution, yet it has been demonstrated to be biologically
active, producing healing effects. The substance becomes homeopathically active only after a process of
vigorous shaking is performed after each dilution. If not,
as you would expect from chemistry, any effect of the
original substance is lost. Why the shaking retains the
pattern of the original substance remains a mystery. It
has been proposed that water molecules are able to
arrange themselves in liquid crystals that could retain a
memory of the original substance and that these crystals
actually multiply when the solution is shaken. This
could account for the fact that the solution as a medicine becomes stronger rather than weaker the more it is
diluted and shaken.

Clinically speaking, the higher the dilution, the
stronger and more long lasting are the effects of the medicine. That means that weaker dilutions (called *high potencies* in homeopathic terms) are stronger medicines.
This concept is paradoxical, and it is homeopathy's
greatest problem in terms of acceptance. People often

cannot believe that homeopathy works until they see the results firsthand. Then they say, "I don't know how or why it works, but it does."

The Willing Suspension of Disbelief

Just for a moment, allow yourself to entertain the possibility that the homeopaths are correct and the chemists are as yet unable to explain why. What would this mean? For one thing, it means that we are dealing with a medicine that is not simply physical and chemical in its nature or its effects. This frees homeopathy from necessarily abiding by the known laws of chemistry and physics and perhaps allows it to inhabit a new territory in scientific thought.

So let's examine some of the facts that are known empirically about the action of homeopathic medicines:

- The healing effect only occurs when the patient's symptoms are similar to symptoms that the substance can cause in healthy people.
- Very small doses can have large effects on a person's health.
- These effects are real, not just a placebo response.
- One dose of medicine can cause a profound healing response lasting for months or years.

Some people may dispute these facts, but a brief examination of the homeopathic literature will prove their veracity. So, just for the sake of argument, accept that these facts might be true and test them for yourself. If you fall and bruise yourself, take a dose of *Arnica montana* 30C. If you have a bee sting, take a dose of *Apis*

30C. You will demonstrate for yourself that homeopathy works. Then try it for the kind of problems covered in this book, such as rage, defiance, and violent behavior, but only under the guidance of an experienced homeopathic practitioner.

7

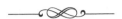

A Different Answer
for Difficult Kids
New Hope for Treating
Defiance and Aggression

Where can parents turn for help with their children who act out, defy them unreasonably, fly into rages, or explode with violent and destructive tantrums? Normal parenting is hard enough, but having to raise a rage-aholic child can be beyond the call of duty. Homeopathy, though not a panacea, offers a viable solution for handling these emotional and behavioral problems that is safe, natural, and highly effective. Homeopathy has the potential to cure children of these distressing states of mind and behavior. Given sufficient time to act and careful attention by an experienced practitioner to medicine selection, dosage, and frequency of medication, homeopathy will produce positive changes in most children. In reviewing our cases, we estimate a 70 percent success rate in children who receive two years of consistent treatment. A significant positive shift often occurs within four to six weeks after taking the medicine, but a minimum of two years of treatment is needed to assure that the improvements are maintained over time.

How Can Homeopathy Help My Child?

Although homeopathy may not work for every child, the majority of our patients have become much less aggressive and violent, considerably nicer, much more compliant, and easier to live with after treatment. They are more capable of dealing with stressful situations, frustration, or simply being told no without losing it and becoming angry, oppositional, aggressive, violent, or destructive. Many children become significantly less reactive and more willing to listen to explanations of what parents want them to do. The ADHD characteristics of distractibility, impulsivity, and hyperactivity become much more manageable (see our book *Ritalin-Free Kids*). Physical fighting with parents, siblings, schoolmates, and friends becomes considerably less frequent. Incidents at school become rare events rather than everyday occurrences. Destruction of property becomes accidental rather than deliberate. Children often develop a greater sense of right and wrong and act as though they now have a conscience that guides their actions, so lying, stealing, and hurting others are considerably diminished.

Does it sound to good to be true? Read the cases in this book, summarized and quoted from our chart notes, and judge for yourself. The stories are presented here just as they were told to us. The results of the homeopathic medicine, good and bad, are there to see. Only the names and other identifying features have been changed. Granted, these are our best cases, some of which seem miraculous, but the results are real. Other cases, not in the book, have been more challenging and the results less astounding. Unfortunately, there are some children whom, try as we might, we cannot help.

With others, though the change is not as immediate or dramatic as the cases in our book, the parents feel that a significant enough change occurs to warrant continued homeopathic treatment. In some of these cases, a dramatic change may not occur for a year or two, when the correct medicine is finally found. Children treated successfully with homeopathy, though not without the ups and downs that occur for every child, can truly be called rage-free kids. Their parents, family members, teachers, and friends can finally go back to living a more normal life.

Why Not Just Use Conventional Medicine?

Conventional treatment of children with behavior disorders is increasingly oriented toward drug therapy, although various forms of counseling, psychotherapy and behavior modification may be used as well. As discussed in the previous chapter, with drugs often come side effects, some simply annoying and some serious, such as tic disorders, or even life-threatening, such as allergic reactions. Most of the side effects, such as appetite loss, insomnia, growth retardation, headaches, and stomachaches, are relatively minor and disappear when the medication is stopped. Unfortunately, for many of these children, the medication cannot be stopped, or serious aggression, destruction, and violence may occur. In fact, the medication may need to be taken for life in order for the person to behave within relatively normal limits and avoid socially unacceptable behavior patterns.

Many parents and children are willing to put up with these side effects, which are much less disruptive

The Advantages of Homeopathic Medicine

- Homeopathic medicine is individualized rather than one-size-fits-all. In fact, homeopathy is based on the individualization of treatment, assuming that each person is unique and needs a medicine that specifically matches his or her pattern of symptoms.
- A well-chosen medicine is highly effective, producing noticeable changes in three weeks to two months after the initial dosing. Progress may continue for many months after the initial effect. In contrast, a dose of conventional medicine only lasts for a few hours.
- Homeopathy is safe and very gentle, with few of the side effects of conventional medication. As you have seen in chapter 5, the pharmaceutical management of rage and defiance has significant potential for side effects, even when it works, and it may only control rather than cure the problem.
- Homeopathy will only change the child's personality for the better. It will not make the child depressed, sleepless, take away her appetite, remove her "spark," or turn the child into a "zombie"—common complaints with conventional medication. An incorrect medicine will generally produce no effect and do no harm.
- Homeopathic medicine is tolerated very well by finicky and oppositional children. It is dissolved in the mouth and tastes good. Many children beg for more. In many cases, one dose can last for months or even for years in some cases.
- Homeopathic treatment may be undertaken as the only mode of treatment or in conjunction with conventional treatment. More frequent dosing may be used for children on conventional medication.

- The cost of homeopathy, which may seem expensive initially because of the time involved in the first visit, is quite economical in the long run. Follow-up visits with the homeopath are infrequent, usually every few months, and generally cost less than a hundred dollars a visit. The medicine, whether given in a single, weekly, or daily dose, rarely costs more than twenty dollars, next to nothing compared with conventional drugs. Homeopathy is not just effective; it is cost-effective as well.
- Homeopathy heals physical as well as mental and emotional problems. Allergies, asthma, digestive problems, infections, childhood illnesses, injuries, and many other health conditions respond well to homeopathic medicine.
- Homeopathy heals and strengthens the whole person, including the immune system, and helps prevent future illness and behavior disorders.

than the rather severe problem behaviors that the medication is controlling. These parents would not even consider going back to the impossible existence that they and their child once endured together before the child was medicated.

Some parents, however, are decidedly uneasy about their child being treated with strong medication with potentially serious side effects. It is a difficult choice to give medication that they believe may harm their child in the long run but that is immediately effective in controlling the child's objectionable, even dangerous behavior. Many parents feel guilty about the trade-off. Other parents simply feel it is a necessary evil or just what you do because it is what the doctor says is necessary to help the child.

When parents are dissatisfied with their doctor's advice, they may be open to an alternative. Homeopathy is not yet mainstream medicine in the United States, although it is well-accepted in other parts of the world, such as England, Germany, France, and India. The willingness to undertake homeopathic treatment requires the abilities to think differently and to accept a medical system whose concepts predate and fly in the face of modern medicine.

It is when conventional medicine does not work, the side effects are too severe, or parents are philosophically opposed to drug treatment that they seek out some other way. Their open-mindedness can lead to a very positive, frequently dramatic, transformation of their child.

Challenges of Homeopathic Treatment

To be fair, homeopathy is not without its challenges. Anyone contemplating homeopathic treatment should be aware of what can happen during the course of treatment. Any competent homeopath, though, is well aware of these situations and trained to manage them. Here are some points to consider:

- Most successful cases are solved within six to twelve months, but even the best homeopath does not always find the correct medicine for a patient, even after months of treatment. Homeopaths vary in methods and experience level. It makes sense to give your practitioner a fair chance to find the medicine before switching to another. It will often be worth the wait. The better your homeopath knows your child and what medicines have already been tried, the more likely she is to find the best medicine. It is also possible, if your homeopath is not having success at finding the medicine to best help your child after nine to twelve months, to request that she consult with someone specializing in your child's particular area of concern.

- Homeopathy is a process, not a one-time event. The homeopath must take an extensive case history and do careful follow-up to see the effects of the medicine in order to decide whether a change is to be made or another dose is required. There may be ups and downs in treatment, some of which may be avoided by consistent follow-through (see chapter 10). This takes commitment on the part of parents and patients alike to stay with the process until the desired results are obtained. Though improvement usually occurs soon after treatment begins, it may take a number of visits over at least one to two years to see all the changes you desire. The parents must be willing to observe their child and report any progress or relapse to the homeopath. The child must be willing to take the medicine and avoid substances that interfere with treatment.

- There may be a period of initial intensification of the child's existing symptoms, which homeopaths call an *aggravation*. This reaction is usually brief but may last several days or even several weeks in some cases. This is not a side effect in the traditional sense but rather a "healing crisis," a natural part of the homeopathic process. It may be unavoidable if healing is to occur. For violent or destructive children, precautions may have to be taken to provide for the safety of the child and others and to protect property from damage.

- In rare cases, symptoms that are part of the symptom picture of the medicine itself, but that are new to the child, may appear. These symptoms are usually minor, short-lived, and disappear if the medication is discontinued.

- Earlier symptoms from the child's health history may appear briefly then disappear, leaving a net improvement in the child's health. This process, called *return of old symptoms,* is a natural part of the homeopathic process and, in fact, is a good sign. We believe it occurs because previous illnesses have left a deep impression in the cellular memory of the individual. It appears that homeopathy has the capacity, when the correct medicine is given, to erase those memories, sometimes permanently.

- Skin eruptions such as rashes, eczema, and warts and discharges of mucus or waste products from the body such as nasal or vaginal discharge or diarrhea may appear for a few days during the healing process. These appearances are also a sign of healing as the body cleanses itself, and usually they go away on their own or, if there is significant discomfort, can be addressed by natural, palliative treatments that are compatible with homeopathy.

The Choice Is Yours

With all of the advantages of homeopathic medicine, it is easy to see why parents all across the United States and Europe are beginning to turn to homeopathy for solutions for ADHD, ODD, CD, Tourette's disorder and other emotional and behavioral problems. When parents realize it is possible to heal all of a child's problems, physical and emotional, with one medicine, and when that medicine is natural, safe, highly effective, and cost-effective, with few if any side effects, many parents are willing to consider homeopathic treatment for their children. Even the challenges involved in homeopathic treatment seem minor when the alternative is using potentially toxic pharmaceutical drugs, sometimes for life.

Our experience, in treating over 1,500 children with ADHD and other behavioral and learning problems, is that homeopathy makes sense for those parents looking for an alternative. For parents who are satisfied with conventional drug therapy from their pediatrician or psychiatrist, there is no need to look any further. Those parents are not usually the ones reading this book. It is the parents who are not happy with conventional treatment and want, or are even desperate for, a better approach. They are the ones who are ready for a different answer for their children.

We are not on a crusade to eliminate conventional psychiatric medication for children, only to provide an alternative that we believe has significant advantages. If what you are already doing makes more sense to you and you are getting good results with an acceptable level of side effects, by all means stay with that kind of treatment. However, if you are ready for an alternative that really works, then read on.

8

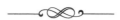

Treating Kids, Not Diagnoses
Individual Treatment
for Unique Children

There is no one in the world exactly like your child. With all of his or her good and bad qualities, no one else has that particular mix of genetics, physical body, environment, and life experience. Why is this point important? Homeopathic philosophy explains that because each person is an individual, he needs an individualized medicine for the best results. Each homeopathic prescription is based on all of the person's symptoms at a given time, which is the complex of his mental and emotional symptoms combined with his specific and general physical symptoms, all of which together is known as the person's *state*. The state is a particular stance in life, with the symptoms that go along with it.

For example, in children who need the medicine *Stramonium,* the stance is similar to a child walking in a dark jungle with imagined danger all around. At any moment a wild animal, monster, or ghost may leap out of the darkness in order to harm her. The child feels a sense of terror and foreboding and longs for light and company. If an individual is actually cornered and attacked in the jungle, she would try to run away or would respond violently to protect herself. A child in a

Stramonium state carries the feeling of the jungle within her, even safe under the covers of her own bedroom. Whenever there is an imagined threat, such as a nightmare or a monster under the bed, she flees to light and the company of her parents or flies into a rage for no apparent reason.

Another child may feel weepy, insecure, and want company but not be in such a drastic state as a child who needs *Stramonium*. The feeling is much less intense and without the strong feelings of terror or the need for violence. Such a child may need *Pulsatilla*, a medicine indicated when the state of those children needing the medicine is a kind of soft, weepy moodiness, constantly changing, with a strong need for love and support. A child matching the state of *Stramonium* may say, "Help! They're trying to get me!" whereas one needing *Pulsatilla* is more likely to entreat, "Please hold me and tell me you love me."

The one homeopathic medicine that best fits the child's symptoms and state will produce the deepest and most long-lasting effect. One person's medicine will not help another person unless they have a very similar state. Ten different children may need ten different medicines, or two children may need the same medicine if they are similar in certain ways that match the picture of the medicine. In conventional medicine, drug therapy is based on the common response of a group of patients to a medication. In homeopathy, it is the unique response of the individual that counts. A person may have no response, a partial response, or a complete healing response when given a homeopathic medicine, depending on the accuracy of the prescription.

In conventional medicine, the physician knows the diagnosis and is familiar with the medicines that have been developed to treat that diagnosis. For depression, for instance, the medicines might be Prozac or Zoloft; for anxiety, Buspar and Paxil. In homeopathy, no matter what the diagnosis, if the homeopath knows the person's unique pattern of symptoms and is able to grasp the individual's state, it is likely that she can select the single medicine that will produce healing. For the homeopath, when the pattern of symptoms is recognized, it functions like a diagnosis for the purpose of selecting the needed medicine.

The Importance of Symptoms

It does not matter whether a person has pneumonia, an allergy to cats, eczema, or conduct disorder; if his symptoms match the homeopathic medicine *Tuberculinum*, only *Tuberculinum* is likely to be extremely helpful. Other homeopathic medicines may act only on the few symptoms that they match but will not have a far-reaching effect. Only the correct medicine will stimulate a full healing response lasting months or years.

Take conduct disorder, for example. Children may be diagnosed with this condition if they have serious antisocial tendencies, aggressive or destructive behavior without the normal restraints of conscience. A homeopath will look at the symptoms of the child and turn them into usable symptoms in the language of the homeopathic literature. Having no conscience may be interpreted as the symptoms "want of moral feeling." Cruelty may be interpreted as the symptom "malicious." Hitting other children may be interpreted as the symptom "striking, in children." Other symptoms that have nothing to do with conduct disorder per se will also be included if they are very strong or intense, such as a desire for oranges, fear of thunderstorms, stomachaches that are better from moving around, or a tendency to sleep on the stomach with the butt up in the air. These symptoms often help differentiate one child with conduct disorder from another. The more unusual, rare, or peculiar the symptoms, the more useful they are for finding an individualized medicine for the child.

All of the child's symptoms are compiled and sorted to see which homeopathic medicines have been known to cure each symptom. Computerized database programs capable of searching the homeopathic literature are often used to aid and speed this process. When a match has been made between the symptoms of the child and the symptoms cured by a particular medicine, further study of the medicine in the homeopathic literature is made to determine the actual suitability of the medicine for this particular child. When the homeopath is satisfied that the match is the best possible, a single homeopathic medicine is prescribed.

Why Not to Prescribe for Your Own Child

How is this medicine chosen? It is best to let a competent, experienced homeopath choose the medicine, rather than choosing it yourself, for a number of reasons. If your child had appendicitis, you would not diagnose it from a book and do the surgery yourself. You would find a competent surgeon who had performed hundreds of operations successfully. The same is true for homeopathy. *Do not prescribe for yourself or your child if you have a serious or chronic condition.* Here is why:

- The homeopath sees many patients with all kinds of different symptom patterns. She learns to differentiate one pattern from many others and can successfully choose the correct homeopathic medicine in most cases. A parent, though knowing his or her child best, usually knows little about homeopathic medicines. It is best to give the homeopath the benefit of your unique knowledge of your child and let her make the decision as to what medicine is best. Try not to second-guess your practitioner but do offer any and all information that may assist the homeopath in understanding your child. We take parents' observations and opinions into account in selecting the medicine, but our experience has been that even if the correct medicine is found by an astute parent, the case still needs careful management to ultimately come to a successful conclusion.

- Parents unfortunately often have difficulty being totally objective about their children, especially parents who are themselves homeopaths. Bias and emotional concerns may cloud their ability to make the proper choice. Suppose the child needs a medicine derived from the tarantula spider. Most parents would not readily admit that their child had characteristics resembling a tarantula, but if the homeopath presents the idea, backed up with sound evidence, the parent may be more willing to go along with the prescription.

- The homeopath needs to objectively evaluate the child's progress after giving the medicine. Although he may want the medicine to be successful just as much as the parents do, it is not his child who is being affected. The homeopath can afford to be more detached about whether the child is improving and how quickly. This approach prevents rash decisions based on the parents' sense of urgency that can spoil the course of treatment, especially if the homeopath is pushed by the parents and makes the wrong decision about treatment.

A competent practitioner will take an accurate and extensive case history from the parents and also interview or observe the child, if possible. From the available information, the homeopath will make the best choice of medicine based on what she knows about the child, verified by the homeopathic literature and her years of experience.

"How Can I Find a Homeopath?"

Many types of medical and lay practitioners practice homeopathy. A growing number of licensed health care practitioners either specialize in homeopathy or prescribe some homeopathic medicines. Other homeopaths, although unlicensed and without formal medical training, can receive certification in homeopathy. Licensing is not always the best way to determine the competence of a homeopath, although it may assure a certain level of medical background and training. If you want a practitioner with some type of medical background, a board-certified homeopath may be your best choice. Those homeopaths who are not medically trained work more as consultants rather than as the child's primary health care provider. What is most important is to find the best-trained and most experienced practitioner who is easy for you to communicate with. Because homeopathic practice is quite challenging, those who do not practice it full-time are less likely to produce the best results. We recommend that you select a practitioner who uses homeopathy in at least 75 percent of his practice.

Training in homeopathy is almost entirely postgraduate and elective through courses and seminars. Because of this, experience, competence and methodology vary widely among practitioners. We urge you to find a *classical* homeopath if you would like to obtain results similar to those in this book. Such a homeopath spends at least an hour in interviewing and observing new patients, prescribes a single homeopathic medicine at a time based on the patient's symptoms, rather than using a machine or muscle testing for diagnosis, and waits at least four to six weeks to evaluate the patient's progress.

For children with serious behavioral problems, it is usually best to find a homeopath who is experienced in treating behavior and attention problems in children. Since this is not always possible, and because homeopaths treat the whole person in any case, find the most experienced practitioner you can, whether in person or through telephone consultations. Since the homeopathic evaluation takes the form of an interview, it is possible to treat children and adults in different cities and countries with considerable success. We have treated children from Latin America, Asia, Russia, Europe, Australia, and other places, often by telephone. These children receive their physical examinations and primary health care from a local provider. Directories of homeopaths are available from organizations listed in the appendix of this book.

9

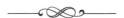

What to Expect from Homeopathic Medicine
The Typical Course of Treatment

The purpose of the homeopathic interview is to collect the information and note the symptoms necessary to find an effective medicine for your child. Everyone concerned, parents and child, is encouraged to tell the child's story in whatever way it comes out spontaneously. The homeopath may ask an open-ended question to get you started and a few questions along the way or just listen, allowing you and your child the space to reveal his or her true nature. Observation is just as important as questioning in the interview, and the homeopath can often learn more by listening than by speaking. A homeopath tries to be attentive to clues about the person's nature, problems, and state from the moment the patient enters the office to the moment she leaves. Little details may be observed that have no importance to anyone but a homeopath looking to see whether a particular pattern will emerge from the dynamics of the interview, the interactions in the waiting room, or on the telephone. A person will usually reveal his state adequately to a good observer and interviewer, leading to an accurate homeopathic prescription.

The homeopath is interested in many aspects of your child's mental and emotional state, behavior, and physical problems. Say whatever comes into your mind about your child: his problems, behavior patterns, your family and his environment, his likes and dislikes, favorite activities, talents and abilities, physical symptoms and illnesses, temperature and weather effects, food cravings and aversions, and whatever makes his symptoms better or worse. Previous psychological testing or laboratory results, reports from the school, and other information are integrated into the verbal interview to round out the picture. You may find your homeopath is not as interested in these types of diagnostic processes as in what your child actually does and how he expresses himself. What is most helpful to the homeopath is absolutely anything about your child that is unusual, strange, out of the ordinary, or out of proportion to his circumstances.

There is a lot to cover in an hour-long interview, but everything that is important is likely to be covered before the interview is finished. You can always call in or send additional information or share it during the next appointment. You may be asked to fill out a medical history form in advance. At or prior to the initial interview, you can ask your homeopath which, if any, previous health or school records are needed.

Helping Your Child Cope with the Interview Process

One of the challenges in treating children with anger, opposition, and other behavioral problems is to gain basic cooperation of the patient herself with the initial and subsequent interviews. Some children are opposed to the interview process simply because their parents want them to do it. Others become bored and restless during the hour or throw tantrums during the interview. Although distracting and disruptive, it is actually helpful for the homeopath to experience your child's real-life behavior, even at its worst.

We typically prefer to interview the parents first, while the child remains occupied with toys or books in the waiting room. This approach gives adolescents an opportunity to chill out and have some space to themselves. It also allows the parents to tell their side of the story truthfully without protestations and constant interruptions from their child and without hurting the child's potentially fragile feelings. Then the child or adolescent can be brought in either with or without the parents. If the parents are absent, he has a chance to tell his part of the story confidentially and without hurting the parents' feelings. If the child would rather be interviewed with the parents present or the parents feel there is no need to speak with the homeopath privately, that is no problem. Each homeopath has his own style of handling appointments.

Spending time alone with the child is particularly important with teenagers. Interviewing a rebellious adolescent and an angry parent together can turn into a "I did not!"–"You did, too!" screaming match. We have found that this can be avoided when we allow the parent to vent first and provide the overall picture of the child and then to spend time with the teenager in private. Adolescents are more likely to want certain information shared with their homeopath to remain confidential. It is also much easier to foster rapport with a teenager on a one-to-one basis, and he is more likely to feel validated and heard. This is especially crucial during the first interview when the tone of the relationship is first established.

The Homeopathic Prescription

At the end of the interview or after a further period of study, your homeopath will prescribe a single homeopathic medicine with the goal of bringing into balance your child's behavior, attention, health, and well-being. The medicine is most often given on a sugar pellet base, dissolved in the mouth. Some homeopaths may give the medicine in liquid form as drops, placed on or under the tongue. The medicine may be given in a single high-potency dose, likely to last for several months or more; in lower-potency doses, designed to be taken more frequently; or in a high-potency dose followed by low-potency doses taken on a particular schedule such as daily or twice a week. Your homeopath will determine the kind of dosing that is best for your child's situation. If your child is not on any other conventional medications, it is likely that a single high-potency dose will be given. High-potency doses are usually given infrequently, generally when symptoms begin to come back after initial improvement.

The Course of Treatment

After the initial prescription, a period of time is allowed in which to observe any changes resulting from the medicine. This is usually four to eight weeks but may be as much as three months. During this time, be aware of shifts in attention, mood, behavior, and attitude. Also note any changes in physical health, including the appearance of any unusual symptoms, rashes, or discharges, as well as changes in appetite, thirst, sleep, and bowel movements. You may notice startling changes and significant transformations, more subtle differences that you have to think about, or no change at all. Ask your child what changes she notices in herself. Be aware of how things are when you start treatment so you can make comparisons with states of health and behavior later on in the course of treatment. Your homeopath keeps detailed notes for comparison. Sometimes when you report little or no change, the homeopath will compare the current situation with the chart notes to make an objective assessment of whether changes have actually occurred.

Although ups and downs may occur in the first two months, if the medicine has acted well, there should be at least a noticeable change in your child's disposition, behavior, and health, beginning in the first six weeks. The first few days or weeks may be rougher than usual. Homeopaths call this a *homeopathic aggravation* or healing crisis. Characteristic symptoms may increase in frequency or intensity, but usually not more than either the child or the parents can endure. Think of it as all the bad behavior being compressed into a short time, allowing the child to be more free of it after that.

Don't be surprised if your normally surly, disobedient, rageful child has suddenly acquired an angelic disposition and a run of perfect behavior, or if she has stopped muttering nasty comments when you get her up in the morning and starts to do her homework for the first time in three years. It's a cause for celebration! No more medicine will be given as long as the momentum

of positive change imparted by the original dose continues. Doses are only given when they are needed. As long
as the patient is improving, his body and mind are allowed to go through the healing process without unnecessary interference.

If at the end of two months, nothing has changed
and nothing has transpired to interfere with treatment
(see the "Do's and Don'ts" sidebar), your homeopath
will retake the case and try to find a better medicine. If
something has definitely interfered with the initial treatment, the original medicine will be given another try before going on to another.

In every case, there are always other options for
medicines if the first medicine fails to act properly. It is
important not to give up on the homeopathic process
entirely if the first medicine does not produce improvement. A number of parents make this mistake out of im-
patience to quickly find a solution for their child's
intolerable behavior problems. A lack of improvement
does not mean that homeopathy will never be effective.
It only means that the first medicine was not sufficiently
similar to your child's symptoms to stimulate a healing
response.

Be patient. Your homeopath will usually find the
correct medicine in the first six months of treatment,
even if one or more medicines does not produce the desired result. Occasionally it takes longer, in complex or
difficult cases, but homeopaths do not give up easily.
We know what wonderful transformations can occur
with the correct medicine and are dedicated to finding
the right medicine for each person. The more the homeopath understands the patient, the sooner the best medicine can be found. Some people are easy to know and
understand; others are more complex. When parents are
able to share clearly what's going on with their child

and what is most unique or out of proportion, it is often possible to select a highly effective medicine even if the child is not terribly disclosive or cooperative.

After the initial prescription, visits are scheduled every few months so that your child's progress can be carefully monitored. Even if your child is doing well, it is important to keep your homeopath informed of any further progress or relapse. A visit or telephone consultation is the best way to do this. It takes at least twenty to thirty minutes of quality interviewing to assess a child's treatment progress and prognosis accurately. When your child is doing well and has shown great improvement, it serves as a good baseline in case things should start going the other way in the future.

It is very difficult for the homeopath to assess the entire process unless she has seen the child at regular intervals, both when the child is doing well and when she is not. If you try to avoid coming for visits out of financial concerns alone, you will shortchange your child and possibly doom the process to failure. If money is a problem, work with your practitioner to find the correct frequency of visits at a price that works for both of you.

Hopefully, the first medicine works and your child does well for months or years. That is the best-case scenario. More often, your child will need several doses of the correct medicine in the first year or so of treatment. With each dose, improvement should occur, so that over time his original problems continue to diminish in frequency and severity. It is important to keep track of your child's progress. If there is any significant relapse after doing better, another dose of medicine should be given to keep up the momentum of improvement. If you wait too long to repeat the medicine, old behaviors can crop up again if the child's state is not yet stably improved.

Do's and Don'ts
for Homeopathic Treatment

There are certain guidelines that can help you
make the most of your child's homeopathic care.
In particular, certain substances and procedures
can interfere with the treatment process. The more
sensitive your child, the more likely these substances can interfere and the best it is to avoid
them entirely. When we say that these can interrupt treatment, we mean that a child whose behavior had improved partially or dramatically may go
back to the way he was prior to treatment after exposure to one of these influences. Although the
medicine can usually be repeated with success, we
recommend the most conservative course, which
is to avoid them entirely throughout the course of
homeopathic treatment. However, it is most crucial
to do so while your homeopath is in the process of
discovering the best medicine for your child. Individual practitioners' recommendations regarding
possible antidotes may vary.

1. DO have your child take the homeopathic medicine exactly as prescribed by your practitioner.
2. DON'T use the following:

   - Coffee (both caffeinated and decaf) and any
     products containing coffee. It is *not* necessary
     to avoid caffeinated beverages unless they
     contain coffee. Chocolate, soda pop, and
     black or green tea are not a problem with
     homeopathy.
   - Products containing strong aromatic sub-
     stances such as camphor, eucalyptus, tea tree
     oil, pine oil, phenol, and menthol. These in-
     clude but are not limited to Ben-Gay, Carmex,
     Blistex, Vick's, Hall's cough drops, Ricola,

Noxema, Chapstick, Tiger Balm, Bag Balm and most liniments, many mouthwashes, and cleaning products such as Lysol and Pine-sol.

- Electric blankets
- Hair permanents
- Dental drilling and ultrasonic cleaning. These procedures may interrupt the action of the homeopathic medicine. If your child needs emergency dental treatment, by all means do it as soon as possible. If the dental work can wait a while, discuss the best timing with your practitioner.

3. DO contact your homeopath if your child has a serious acute illness. Books on acute homeopathic care such as our *Homeopathic Self-Care: The Quick and Easy Guide for the Whole Family* can be helpful. Your homeopathic practitioner may want you to consult a medical doctor, but it is best to inquire first so as to maximize your child's homeopathic care. If your child has a medical emergency, seek help from a qualified medical professional immediately.

4. DO keep in touch with your homeopath about significant changes in your child's condition. Make appointments at intervals suggested by your practitioner for follow-up care.

5. DO continue with the homeopathic process until you have achieved the desired results with your child. Work closely with your homeopath to get your child's needs met in the best way possible.

10

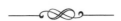

How to Cope with Your Challenging Child
Survival Strategies for Families

The trick here is to separate your child's actions from who he is as a person. You have probably heard of the idea that you can love someone even if you don't like what they have done. In other words, you can disapprove, mildly or strongly, of the behavior without blanketly disapproving of the child. There is no stronger glue than love. Let your child know that, no matter what he has done, you are in his corner and will be there to love, support, and encourage him.

Lett your kid know that you are always there for him. Again, this is not to say that you will give permission for or encourage everything he wants to do but to support him to make the best possible choices and, if he doesn't, to learn from his mistakes.

Don't Be Afraid to Discipline Your Child

Children need to know boundaries. The adults that we have seen who never felt they were given clear boundaries or guidelines as youngsters frequently have problems knowing who they are and where they stand as adults. Make sure the rules are fair and clear and there is a consequence to breaking them. If a child knows that the rules are not only in her best interest but for the good of everyone involved, that the rules exist for a good reason, she will be more likely to follow them. And when your child does something really dangerous or really bad, make it perfectly clear that her behavior is not acceptable and that you still love her.

Be Consistent

Whatever rules or guidelines you establish for your child, be consistent. Don't give mixed messages. Set realistic and reasonable limits and stick to them. If your child thinks he can walk all over you, he will. If he respects you, he is likely to respect his teachers, friends, and others around him. Consistency may be a challenge in divorced or blended families, but do your best to keep expectations clear.

Make the Punishment Fit the Crime

Kids need to learn the difference between right and wrong and to face the consequences of their actions. But those consequences should be appropriate, not excessive. We treated one young boy in the Midwest whose mom washed his mouth out with soap whenever he talked back to her. We tried to tactfully broach the subject of excessive punishment. That's what her mother had done to her, and she figured she ought to do the same.

What's most important is that your child appreciate what he's done, how he could have acted differently, and learn to make better choices in the future. Learn what types of consequences make the most impact on your child with the least pain. Then use them sparingly. This approach will be much more effective than constant time-outs or taking away his Nintendo every other day. If you're having to punish your child on a regular basis, take a closer look at your parenting and at your child.

Catch Your Kid Doing Something Right

We remember going to a lecture by Elizabeth Kübler-Ross, who demystified the stages of dealing with death and dying. She told the story of a young man who had a habit of leaving his clothes all around the house. It drove his mom crazy. Then one day he died in a motor-cycle accident. From that time the house seemed too darned clean to his mom. She wished every day that he were still around to mess it up.

Kids are on a steep learning curve, and they make lots of mistakes in the process—such as falling over and over again before they learn to walk. You may feel that there is lots to criticize and little to praise. Be vigilant, and every time you see your kid doing something great or creative or thoughtful, tell her how wonderful she is, how much you love her, and how glad you are to be her mom or dad.

Praise, Praise, Praise

Glen Pearson, a Dallas psychiatrist, claims that "maintaining a positive learning environment minimizes the need for punishment." He urges parents to think about behavior in three categories: desirable, completely unacceptable, and annoying. "The correct response is to lavish praise on the first, impose swift and sure punishment on the second and utterly ignore the third."[1]

Positive reinforcement is always more effective in producing the desired result than criticism, blame, and punishment. We all like to feel good about ourselves, and your child is no exception. Make it a practice to give your child at least one compliment every day. If you like your kid, this will be easy. If you don't, this approach will, over time, help you to see the best in him and to feel more positive and loving.

Keep Your Child Safe but Not Too Safe

As is obvious from many of the newspaper reports that we cite in our book, the world is not always a safe place, and bad things do happen to good people. Be cautious, and do whatever is necessary to teach your child safety—whatever is appropriate for where you live, where she goes to school, and when she might be unsupervised. But don't teach your child to be paranoid. We recently spoke with an adult who was taught by her Holocaust-surviving parents that the world was a dangerous place and she might be apprehended at any moment. This message penetrated her psyche so deeply that she lives in constant fear to this day that something dreadful might happen to herself or her son. Their intentions were to protect their precious child; instead they taught her to live in a prison.

Violence Does Not Solve Violence

At times your child's rage may drive *you* to rage. Kids have a knack for knowing just where to push their parents liftoff buttons. You may feel like striking back at your child, but it won't work, at least not for very long. If you are tempted to physically hurt your child, get help. It is normal to feel irritated, impatient, and angry. But if these emotions predominate or are frequent, do whatever is necessary to get a handle on your own emotions so that you, too, are rage-free.

Use any techniques that work for you to learn to manage your child's aggression without becoming aggressive yourself. These may include taking parenting or anger management classes, reading books on these topics, pursuing psychotherapy, or becoming a homeopathic patient yourself.

Be an Example for Your Child

Take an active role in supporting, guiding, and encouraging him in every area of his life. Know how he is doing in school, where he goes, who his friends are, and what makes him tick. Be an example to him, a model of how you would like him to act. If you want an honest child, be honest yourself. It's funny how much kids turn out like their parents. Some of the most kind and compassionate kids in our practice are those whose parents volunteer to help the poor or open their hearts to others in love and generosity.

Develop a Strategy

First, take an inventory of what is and isn't working for your family as a unit. Be specific. Second, talk about it with your child to get her perspective. Does she agree? If it's not working for you, then maybe it's not working for her, either. Then, if possible, set goals together and agree on a reasonable course of action. If you cannot reason with your child, this is something you will need to brainstorm with your partner or your child's teacher or appropriate health professional.

Change Behavior in Small Steps

Once you have embarked on a strategy, remember that change is often incremental. Take one step at a time. Transformation is usually an ongoing process. Be satisfied with steady improvement. Evaluate your child's progress every month or two rather than every day. That way you are likely to be pleasantly surprised at how much he has changed. Then be sure to tell him about it.

Choose Your Battles Carefully

Very few things are worth fighting about, especially with kids. Pick the big ones, the life-or-death issues that are most crucial. You may even want to list them in order of greatest to least importance. Perhaps his lying to you about missing school is a big one. But his sneaking the third chocolate chip cookie may fall under the "not important" category. It will be far easier to hold your ground on those issues about which you feel very strongly. and your home will be a lot more peaceful.

Talk to Your Child Often

Next to love, the most important thing in raising a child is open communication. It is vital that your child know she can always come to you to talk about anything—that nothing is taboo. If you share your own thoughts, feelings, and reasoning, you teach your child to do the same. You want her to come to you first with her important questions or concerns about life rather than to go to someone who may not necessarily give her the best advice. Ask her what she thinks, wonders, and dreams about without being invasive. Then perhaps you can have one of those relationships where you aren't just parent and child but also friends.

Respect Your Child

Your child is a one-of-a-kind, special, and highly valuable human being—not identical to you or anyone else. She has her own ideas, creativity, and spirit. Feed and nurture your child's individuality. Respect her comments, perceptions, feelings, and needs even if you did not agree with them. Your child is like a plant that you carefully planted in the ground, watered, and bathed in sunlight. Now you can watch that plant grow, flourish, blossom, and bear fruit. Your child is one of your greatest contributions, if not *the* greatest, to the world.

Have Regular Family Meetings

A family meeting is an opportunity, perhaps on a weekly basis, for everyone in the family to sit down together and share their needs and concerns. Each member of the family has a chance to speak uninterrupted. It's a time to hear each other out in a respectful, caring atmosphere. You'll need to set ground rules so that the meetings don't turn into ongoing, heated debates.

Whenever appropriate, make decisions as a family so that everyone feels heard and included.

Challenge Your Child to Learn and Grow

Provide an atmosphere that encourages your child to inquire, explore, discover, and satisfy his curiosity. Find out what excites and inspires your child. Then seek out opportunities to feed his inquiring mind. If he loves dinosaurs, exhaust the resources of the library so that he can learn everything he wants to know about them. Take him to museums, plays, concerts, anywhere that catches his learning fancy. If he takes the lead, be right there behind him. If he lags behind, encourage him to learn all that he can learn and be all that he can be.

Find the best possible educational setting (and there are many) for your unique child. Whether public or private, alternative or home school, different children thrive in different learning environments.

Have Fun with Your Kid

One of the most delightful thing about kids is that, through them, the rest of us can be kids again, too. There is nothing like the light-hearted spirit of a happy child to brighten up your day. Sure, some kids are like storm clouds, but hopefully the next day will be brighter and clearer for them. Whether it is visiting the aquarium, flying a kite, blowing bubbles, taking a bike ride, romping on the beach, or accompanying your child to his favorite movie, enjoy him while he's still a child. They grow up way too fast.

Get Help When You Need It

If you feel that you are in over your head, ask for help—help for your child and for yourself, too. Tap your community for support. It may be a child psychiatrist, family therapist, rabbi or minister, or a homeopath. Perhaps a support group, a twelve-step program, or a Big Brother program can offer relief and assistance. Parenting is a challenging job with any child, much less a difficult one. Special funding and programs are available for special-need children. Take advantage of these resources, and admit when you can't handle it all by yourself.

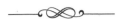

11

The More Help, the Better
For Teachers and
Juvenile Justice Professionals

The lives of teachers used to be much simpler: preparing teaching materials, developing lesson plans, assigning homework, giving and grading tests, attending parent-teacher conferences, turning in report card grades. Now teachers have the biggest responsibility of all: staying alive and making sure their students do the same. Not that every classroom is a potential battlefield. It's just that kids can be unpredictable, and, as we've seen in Springfield, Oregon, Jonesboro, Arkansas, and elsewhere, you just don't know what will happen next. The classroom and school grounds can also be unpredictable.

A case in point is the youngster mentioned recently in our local newspaper:

> When he was in the first grade, he was kicked out of school for stabbing his principal with a pencil. Since then, the Seattle sophomore has been in 17 schools and 20 foster homes. He has trouble sleeping at night because he thinks of how he misses his mother, whom he hasn't seen since second grade. When he's awake in the middle of the night, he

sometimes writes to his ex-girlfriend about death and dying and anger. He has thought about getting a gun from his uncle's room and using it to kill his father, who he fears will take away his 4-year-old brother. There may be no students more challenging to teach than those who, like this youth, are classified as seriously behaviorally disturbed (SBD). More than 5,000 have been identified around the state [of Washington].[1]

SBD children, the article continues, are typically the students who, when they are able enough to remain in regular classrooms, are referred to as the "bad kids" or "losers" because of their aggressive and disruptive behavior and poor academic performance. More than half of these kids fail to graduate from high school. "And the later the student's disability is diagnosed, the worse the prospect of graduation," warns Gene Edgar, a professor of education at the University of Washington who has been studying SBD students for 30 years. "Of all special-education students, SBD students, seventy-five percent of whom are males, have the worst graduation rate and poorest success rate after high school," reports Tom Hanley, an education-research analyst at the U.S. Department of Education.[2]

It can be a challenge to keep the kids in the classroom from becoming bored stiff while educating them and keeping everyone safe.

One elementary school teacher in Massachusetts exercised questionable judgment and unintentionally become a advocate for potential violence. He gave children altered lyrics to "Rudolph the Red-Nosed Reindeer" in which Santa asks a gunman to shoot his wife. The lyrics were included in a packet of Christmas songs handed out to children in which the song was renamed "Deadeye the Two-Gun Slinger." The words were changed to: "Then one foggy Christmas Eve, Santa came to say, 'Deadeye with your gun so bright, won't you shoot my wife tonight?'" The school superintendent reprimanded the teacher, but felt that an apology or explanation to the children would compound the mistake.[3]

A Few Words to Teachers About Homeopathy

There is no one answer for every child or family. This is a country of diversity in nearly every aspect of our society, and health care is no different. We ask you to keep an open mind as you attempt to give children the best education and optimal classroom environment. You will find disruptive and challenging children whose parents are completely in favor of conventional medications and who respond to them very well. In this situation the parents, teacher, and hopefully the child will all be satisfied. Others do not do well with prescription medications. Either they suffer from side effects, or they are no longer themselves. Perhaps they can't gain weight, or their parents see them turn into robots or zombies. In some cases, it's as if the child's spirited nature is lost. With other children, the conventional medications, no matter how many are tried, do not produce meaningful and lasting results. Or the parents of the child may be oriented toward alternative medicine and choose not to medicate their children.

Yes, you are the teacher and you have a responsibility to maintain a positive learning environment in your classroom. But we ask you to not put too much pressure on parents too quickly and to respect their beliefs while considering the possibility that natural medicine may work wonders with the problem child in your class. Read this book and others to learn what new and alternative approaches are available. Pediatricians and psychiatrists will readily admit that they don't have a magic bullet for violent and aggressive children.

If one of your students is receiving homeopathic treatment, please observe that child so you can provide helpful feedback to the parents. We find the reports of teachers, counselors, and school psychologists invaluable in assessing how much progress a child is making with homeopathy. One other request that may seem a bit strange to you involves making sure the child avoids particular substances that can interfere with homeopathic treatment. If such exposures—to Lysol or Pinesol, for example—occur in your classroom, the parents might request that you use an alternative product.

Kids with significant behavior problems can ruin everybody's learning experience and good time. The more we can work together to help find answers for these children, the better.

Innovative Educational Programs

In our research, we came across two particular programs that we found to be especially inspiring and would like to make you aware of them. Horizon House, established in 1964 as a school for emotionally disabled children in Charleston County, South Carolina, works with the kids that have failed everywhere else. They may be hyperactive, depressed, psychotic, abused, children of alcoholic or drug-abusing parents, or juvenile delinquents. Their goal is to mainstream as many of their students as possible. Their philosophy: "By the time students are referred here, we simply cannot allow them to fail." Teachers, counselors, and aides come to Horizon House to teach the kids who have exhausted everyone else's patience. The effort seems to be paying off. "The latest Horizon House studies show about 70 percent of students make it back to their home schools for another chance. They come back to visit from time to time as police officers, electricians, plumbers, and insurance salesman to say 'Thanks.'"[4]

The Fairfax County, Virginia, school district is taking a different approach to assisting troubled students by training regular classroom teachers and principals in dealing with and relating to troubled and disruptive children. The intensive ninety-hour in-service training, which includes watching videos on youth gangs, seems to be making an impact. By the end of the class, educators are often able to see their students in a new light and to have a much greater chance of helping them turn their lives around.[5] By better understanding how children at risk think and why they behave as they do, educators are in a much better position to help them.

There are undoubtedly many other programs around the country attempting to transform the lives of children and adolescents in a positive way. Efforts like these may take a great deal of vision and hard work, but the long-term rewards are well worth it.

Juvenile Delinquency

Once a disturbed or disruptive child, by committing acts of vandalism, theft, assault, or other crimes, has entered the legal system, he is treading a dangerous path. In many cases, these youths suffer from serious mental and emotional problems. At least 150,000 youths in the juvenile justice system are estimated to have at least one diagnosable mental disorder. "Often children enter the juvenile justice system because they haven't gotten adequate mental health treatment," says Regina Hicks, deputy of child and adolescent services for Harris County Mental Health Mental Retardation Authority [MHMR]. "Within the offender population you can have major mental illness, antisocial kids, a whole conglomerate of different types of children who have done the same acts."[6]

The number of serious crimes committed by preadolescent children is mind-boggling. When an act is unconscionable and destructive to property or, more important, human lives, it is difficult for all involved to know how to find the best solution to a terrible situation. Should these kids be treated according to their ages or to the degree of their crime? The [Washington] State Supreme Court responded to this dilemma by making it easier for authorities to prosecute children, ages 8 through 11, who commit crimes. The court decided that prosecutors only have to show the child understood the nature of the act and knew the act was wrong.[7]

An Alternative to Incarceration?

Is jail or prison the long-term answer for these youngsters? A First Time Offenders Program funded by the Texas state legislature offers treatment to young offenders with a psychiatric diagnosis such as depression or con-duct disorder. Focusing on parent training and anger management, 90 percent of children in the program have been able to avoid a second arrest. Pre- and post-treatment evaluations show that 73 percent improved in their school behavior.

Another progressive program in Texas, the Burnett Bayland Reception Center, emphasizes a thorough as-sessment of the educational and mental health needs of youth before placement in a probationary youth pro-gram such as boot camp. It also offers expanding treat-ment options. Hopefully, this new facility, combined with a significant drop in violent crime by juvenile offenders nationwide, will increase the number of chil-dren tested from the mere 1,500 annually out of approx-imately 25,000 minors arrested each year in Harris County alone.[8]

We believe that these disturbed children need to be treated as individuals. It is important to assess as thor-oughly as possible what went wrong in their lives. What led them to make the detrimental choices that they did? Whether the cause is mental illness, abuse, or some-thing entirely different, it is essential to evaluate whether these kids can be truly rehabilitated in any way. Clearly potential future victims of these children need to be protected, but what a waste to throw away these valuable human lives.

An Invitation to the Juvenile Criminal Justice System

We wonder whether there is some way that homeo-pathic medicine can be used within the criminal justice system to benefit some of these lost souls, such as the prisoner we mentioned earlier who wrote to us for help from a state penitentiary. Given some of the positive results that we and other homeopaths have seen with disturbed children, perhaps a pilot program could be established to evaluate the efficacy of homeopathic medicine with this population. There is little to lose and much to potentially gain.

12

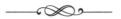

Let's Put Our Heads Together
For Physicians, Psychologists, and Other Mental Health Professionals

Middle America has dabbled in alternative care since the 1970s. But as Harvard researchers reported in JAMA's (*Journal of the American Medical Association*) lead article, the trend has exploded during the '90s. By comparing their new survey results with earlier ones, the researchers showed that reliance on alternative practitioners, from hypnotists to homeopaths, has grown by nearly 50 percent during the 1990s.[1]

"What, then," ask the authors in a *Newsweek* article on the alternative medicine boom, "distinguishes 'alternative' from 'mainstream' medicine?"

Alternative practitioners have been known to put belief before evidence—but so have conventional physicians. As Dr. James Dalen writes in the current *Archives on Internal Medicine*, fewer than half of the protocols now used to prevent blood clots in people with cardiovascular disease have been evaluated in controlled clinical trials. Yet no one calls the untested ones unconventional. "In my opinion," he writes, "the principal distinguishing characteristic of unconventional and conventional therapies is their source of introduction . . . American academic medicine has a bias against outsiders."[2]

Granted, as naturopathic physicians board certified in homeopathic medicine, we are definitely in the outsider category (and proud of it). We do believe, however, that we and other homeopaths can make a significant contribution to the health care system. It has been over twenty years since we entered naturopathic medical school. Hardly anyone had even heard of the type of medicine we were studying back then. Now, thanks to consumer demand for health professionals offering natural alternatives, the establishment of the Office of Alternative Medicine (recently renamed the National Center for Complementary and Alternative Medicine), the growing interest in research, and the large number of students clamoring to study alternative and complementary medicine, our type of medicine is no longer in the closet. The surge of enthusiasm about the popular movie *Patch Adams* demonstrates the paradigm of treating patients as people with feelings as well as bodies. This concept is so attractive that Patch's hospital, although the construction is not even completed, has a waiting list of over a thousand medical students and health care providers.

As physicians, psychologists, and mental health professionals, you are likely to have patients or clients who are using alternative medicine or even using it yourself. Whether or not you are specifically familiar with homeopathy, you are undoubtedly aware of the trend toward natural medicine and therapies. We hope that you will read our book with an open-minded curiosity about how what we have to share may help some of the children that are not responding to your current treatment.

Homeopathic Medicine
Is Gaining Acceptance Worldwide

As mentioned briefly in our introductory material about the prevalence of homeopathy, this form of medicine is widely used in many parts of the world, especially Europe. Referrals to homeopathic physicians and practitioners are commonplace. Over 42 percent of British family practitioners refer to homeopaths.[3] Not only do eleven thousand French physicians prescribe homeopathic medicines themselves, as dispensed by more than twenty thousand pharmacies, but up to 70 percent of conventional physicians in France, although they may not practice homeopathy, accept it as a form of medicine.[4] The national health care systems of Britain and France offer coverage of homeopathic practitioners. The United States is just beginning to catch up.

A Growing Body of Homeopathic Research

The main criticism of homeopathic medicine among conventional medical practitioners is that there's nothing in the medicines and they don't work. The truth is that homeopathic medicines are meticulously regulated by the FDA and, as mentioned in chapter 6, that considerable research has already been conducted on homeopathy. We all agree that more studies are needed in a variety of areas on the efficacy of homeopathic medicine; however, it is an erroneous belief that no research has been done to date. There are well over one hundred documented studies of the effectiveness of homeopathy, a number of which are double-blind (see chapter 6). If your time is limited and you can only read one, we recommend "Are the Clinical Effects of Homeopathy Placebo

Effects? A Meta-Analysis of Placebo-Controlled Trials" published in the esteemed British medical journal *Lancet*.[5]

Homeopathy Is Effective in Treating Mental and Emotional Problems

Before attending naturopathic medical school, we worked in the trenches of the mental health system ourselves in both inpatient and outpatient settings with a varied population. We appreciate the spectrum of individuals with mental and emotional problems, what they need, and what conventional medicine has to offer. Our search for a safer, highly effective natural alternative to psychiatric medications led us to homeopathy. We have always been extraordinarily impressed with the results of homeopathy when compared with conventional psychiatric treatment. We are not talking about simply mediocre clinical results but significant and often dramatic improvements, even in patients, children and adults, who have suffered from their symptoms for a number of years. These results are obtained without the side effects of most conventional medications. In fact there is no need for a homeopathic PDR (*Physician's Desk Reference*) because the side effects common to many psychiatric medications are relatively nonexistent with homeopathic medicines.

Homeopathy Is the Epitome of Whole-Person Medicine

The very nature of homeopathic case taking, case analysis, and prescription entails taking into consideration not just one or two but *all* of the individual's symptoms.

This does not mean giving one medicine for defiance and rage and a second for recurrent otitis media (ear infections), asthma, or chronic headaches. We, as homeopaths, want to learn everything we possibly can about the child so that we can understand what made him the way he is at as deep a level as possible. When a homeopathic medicine is correctly chosen, not some but *all* of these symptoms should improve. Such overall healing is the result of helping the person to become balanced at a fundamental level rather than merely treating the person superficially or symptom by symptom. On the practical level with a child, this means only one medication at a time, given infrequently. The simplicity of the treatment increases patient compliance and decreases the cost of medications.

Conventional Medicine Offers No Easy Solution for Aggressive Behavior

For those interested in pharmaceutical solutions, orthodox medicine has much to offer for ADHD and depression. There is no doubt that stimulant medications such as Ritalin and Adderall have significant effects on attention, restlessness, and impulsivity in many children. The new generation of antidepressants, SSRIs such as Prozac, have helped many adults and some children alleviate depression and cope with a number of other conditions. However, when we talk about aggression without ADHD, or prominent symptoms such as seizures or depression that might lead to a variety of medications, it is another story. Selecting the appropriate conventional medicines for angry kids is generally a matter of trial and error. Given how intractable many of these difficult children are to treat, it makes sense to explore another treatment option that could produce significant benefits.

You Are Likely to Have Patients/Clients Requesting Alternative Medicine

Given the growing trend in the United States toward alternative medicine and the popularity of books such as ours that educate the public about the widespread benefits of homeopathic medicine, it is likely that some of your patients or clients will ask you about natural alternatives for their children and themselves. In fact, if you are not being asked about it, some of your patients are probably doing it on their own and are hesitant to say anything about it to you. When we first started practicing homeopathy, it was much more common for medical doctors to warn their patients about the possible harm of choosing alternative medicine over conventional treatment. Now the response, in the case of an open-minded physician, is more likely to be, "Whatever you're doing seems to be working, so don't change a thing" or "If you think it will work for you, by all means try it" or "Tell me the name of that medicine that helped you so I can read about it for myself."

How to Refer to a Specialist in Homeopathy

Washington state, where we practice, happens to be the most progressive of all the states in terms of insurance reimbursement for alternative health care, thanks in large part to our pioneering and outspoken insurance commissioner, Deborah Senn. All licensed health care providers, including medical doctors, osteopaths, naturopathic physicians, chiropractors, acupuncturists, midwives, and massage therapists, are covered in some form in Washington. Although the largest insurers have tried to fight providing these services to their customers, the U.S. Supreme Court recently threw out their appeal, guaranteeing that coverage for all licensed practitioners will continue to be available in Washington.

In most cases, those homeopathic practitioners covered by third-party payors are considered specialists; however, some may be covered as primary care practitioners. If you wish to refer to homeopaths who have been board certified, your options are practitioners with a designation of DHANP (diplomate of the Homeopathic Academy of Naturopathic Physicians) or DHt (doctor of homeotherapeutics). Both the Council for Homeopathic Certification and the North American Society of Homeopaths offer examinations, primarily to unlicensed homeopathic practitioners. The number of qualified homeopaths in the United States is steadily growing. You can consult the appendix of this book for specific referral information.

What We Recommend in This Book Will Not Interfere with Your Treatment

Homeopathic medicines do *not* interfere with conventional medications. Most practitioners will work in conjunction with the medications that the patient is already taking. However, it is common for the practitioner to recommend that, as the patient improves, he or his parents consult with you about decreasing the dosage of or discontinuing the prescription medications. We have found that many physicians and psychologists, particularly in the case of children, are only too happy to stop the medicine once they are convinced that homeopathic medicine has produced a significant improvement.

The same is true for psychotherapy. Homeopathy cannot undermine or dilute what you are accomplishing with your client in therapy. To the contrary, the angry child treated successfully with homeopathy will become less angry, more able to reason, and will develop a conscience if he lacked one before treatment. It will make your job as a psychotherapist easier and is likely to reduce the duration of treatment.

Working Together to Transform the Lives of Challenging Kids

Let's join forces to provide these children with the best of the conventional and alternative worlds. You do what you do best and let homeopaths do so, too. After all, it is much more important to help people become free of their suffering than to prove which approach is "right." And, given that no one therapeutic modality works for everyone, our patients and clients will be the ones to gain, and we can all learn a great deal in the process.

True Stories from Our Clinical Practice: Homeopathic Successes with Defiant, Aggressive, and Violent Kids

13

Temper Tantrums in Toddlers and Beyond
A Rough Beginning

The term aggression covers a whole range of acts that vary according to age-typical manifestations, severity, and choice of opponents or victims. Thus, aggression is not a unitary term but consists of different manifestations, including verbal aggression, bullying, physical fighting, and different forms of violence, such as robbery, rape, and homicide.[1]

But aggression can begin way before children are capable of any of these actions and even before they have the ability to talk. "The earliest manifestations of aggression occur in the infant's earliest encounters with the social world." Most infants show signs of frustration and rage; particular facial gestures associated with the experience of anger in adults can be identified as early as three months of age.[2]

Kids will be kids, and babies will fuss and cry. Yet what homeopaths look for is attitude or behavior out of the ordinary for that child's particular set of circumstances. A baby who cries when she needs to have her diaper changed, when she's ready to nurse, or when

she's left alone is perfectly normal. One who cries practically all the time except when she is being held is not.

Never Too Young to Tantrum

Marie had been a patient of ours for six years and had
been helped a lot with her chronic allergies. It took her
a year and a half to get pregnant. We reassured her
many times not to worry, that her chances of becoming
pregnant within two years were very good. "Being a
mom is all I want to do right now!" Marie lamented.
Nature took its course, and Maria did give birth to a
bundle of joy, but she soon discovered that motherhood
was not all bliss. She called in desperation when Tricia
was only two weeks and three days old. The little baby
was miserable with gas. She grunted and moaned and
strained to have a bowel movement. Each episode
lasted thirty to sixty minutes. It took Tricia ten to fifteen
minutes to burp after each feeding. Marie had found it
too painful to nurse and was giving the baby a bottle.
Tricia's pediatrician was unable to help. We recommended goat's milk supplemented with folic acid, but
Marie was unable to find it in her area. Tricia seemed to
experience tremendous relief after burping or having a
bowel movement. Marie noticed that the baby's abdomen felt hard as a rock. We gave the baby a dose of
Carbo vegetabilis (vegetable charcoal) and the colic
went away. Charcoal, whether in homeopathic or
herbal form, is well known to relieve gas. Since homeopathic medicines are sweet and prepared in the form of
tiny pellets, they are quite palatable and easy to admin-
ister, even in newborns.

We next heard from Marie seven weeks later. Tricia had turned into a fussy nine-week-old. She was now demanding her mom's attention twenty-four hours a day. The baby never wanted to be alone. She needed to know her mother was present at all times. Tricia was very particular about how she wanted to be attended to, or else she screamed, day or night. She had to be carried facing outward with her mom's hand on her tummy or chest. Being carried on her back with her head looking over Marie's shoulder absolutely wouldn't do.

Tricia was rarely content. Even though less than two months old, she appeared to be easily bored. It angered her when she couldn't get her tiny hands into her mouth fast enough. Tricia was so fussy when her mother left the room that Marie's showers were now limited to two minutes. The only thing that consoled the infant was a bottle, but she was satisfied to suck for only a few minutes. Marie fed her every two hours, more often if she was really upset. Tricia seemed frustrated nearly all of the time.

This baby was very alert for her age. She was a mover and a kicker. Easily upset when she couldn't have her way, she hated the stroller and demanded to be carried around in a front pack. Later, she had no tolerance for the pack and insisted on being wheeled in the stroller. Initially she loved her pacifier. Now she hated it. Tricia had to have everything exactly how she wanted it. Otherwise she flailed her arms and legs, clenched her fists, and squeezed her eyes closed tightly. Even her little lips quivered with anger. The little angel had rapidly turned into a big handful. Tricia's pediatrician remarked, "Wow! You've got a really fussy baby!"

A week earlier Tricia had begun to drool profusely. Marie noticed a hard, white area on her gum. She was told the baby was too young for teething, but all indications pointed to that conclusion. And Marie, a young, new mom, was wondering whether she had chosen the wrong career.

The most common medicine for fussy, tantrummy babies, and the one that helped Tricia, is *Chamomilla* (chamomile). It is often associated with fussiness during teething, especially when the child screams inconsolably and only seems comforted by being carried or rocked. The discomfort is so extreme that the babies can literally shriek for hours on end.

One dose of *Chamomilla* was all that was needed to turn things around for the better. Marie called three weeks later to say that Tricia was not nearly so fussy. When we spoke with Marie recently, Tricia was four months old. She was now sleeping six to seven hours a night. Marie rated the overall improvement to be 60 to 70 percent. She was a lot happier and was feeding five to six times a day instead of every one and a half to two hours. No teeth had broken through yet. Thanks to the *Chamomilla,* both mother and baby were much more content. Now Tricia is ten months old. We just spoke with her relieved mom, who assured us that Tricia is sleeping through the night, teething without hysterical screaming or even obvious discomfort, and gets upset only when she wants something she can't have. Now Tricia is indeed the bundle of joy Marie had longed for so fervently.

Not an Easy Baby

The next story is about a prickly baby, the first child and first grandchild of a doting Jewish family, one of the most calm, warm, and loving families we have ever met.

Claudia and her husband just assumed their little girl would fit right into the family. So much for assumptions with kids.

Claudia was another woman who had been helped tremendously with homeopathy for her musculoskeletal problems, and now she wanted us to treat her daughter. Even Claudia, a remarkably patient and loving woman, described Christy as "not an easy baby." First the child had thrush and the mom suffered from mastitis, so nursing became a painful proposition. Claudia persisted through the discomfort. Then came the ear infections. The antibiotics prescribed by Christy's pediatrician caused a vaginal yeast infection. When the family moved out of state, we did not hear from Claudia for almost two years.

Claudia phoned us again when Christy turned two and a half. She had been treated by a local homeopath for a year without success, mainly for vaginal pain and bladder infections. Christy had recently begun to exhibit temper tantrums. "She's sassy and demanding. She'll instruct me, 'No! Don't do that!' Or 'Stay away.' When she's frustrated, she orders me or her grandparents to do or get what she wants. She doesn't warm up to people very easily. Christy has wonderful, affectionate grandparents. They feel hurt when she keeps them at a distance and fights being picked up. She even turns her head away from her dad when he tries to kiss her. Even being looked at upsets her."

Christy feared dogs and the dark. She was starting to be aggressive, which was pretty shocking to her calm, gentle parents. When a younger child bothered her, she responded with a whack. Sometimes she hit other children without any cause. A cautious child, she did not like performing in front of others but sang out loud in bed for forty-five minutes before falling asleep. She loved to dance, jump, and be outside. Christy was more of an observer than a participant, both around people and animals, and initiated contact only on her own terms.

Mercurius solubilus (mercury) produced some positive results. Christy acted out less verbally, her tantrums became less frequent, and she didn't order others around as much. But her behavior was still disturbing to her parents, including slapping another child across the face or striking out at younger kids. The vacuum cleaner was a new addition to her list of fears. She still didn't want her parents to kiss her unless she asked them to. Christy was now dancing all day long. Her vaginal yeast infection had returned. We prescribed the *Mercurius* in a higher potency.

By the time of the next visit, Christy had turned three. Her behavior had taken a turn for the worse at a week-long family reunion where she slugged her cousins, grabbed at their faces, and was generally impossible to be around. Claudia was so mortified that she tried to book an earlier flight, but all the flights were full. Matters were made worse by the fact that Christy now had a baby brother. "On the way to the supermarket today," Claudia recounted, "she screamed for me to put the baby down and hold her instead. Then she ordered me to remove her from the car."

Sibling rivalry caused Christy's belligerence to escalate. She had resorted to biting her mother or herself. As she writhed on the floor, shrieking, "No, you can't!" it was as if she sunk her teeth into something to get any relief from her misery. Not only did she hit and grab, but now she scratched other children's faces as well. She even woke from sleep screaming, "No!"

The only thing that made Christy happy was to dance. And dance she did, all day long. Her face showed pure delight at she moved her body and bounced her head to the beat. Best of all was to dance naked: "Let's take off our pants and dance!" Much more restless than ever before, anytime she had a chance, she climbed, jumped, and flung her body. The rudeness with strangers persisted. She still acted in a guarded fashion with everyone but her mom. She was terrified of dogs but loved bread.

Now the symptoms were so out of proportion that the medicine required was obvious. A rude, restless, aggressive child who loves to dance, jump, climb, and sing is an indication for *Tarentula* (tarantula spider). They love to dance, rock, and tap rhythmically and can work themselves up into a frenzy.

The change was impressive. When we spoke with Claudia one month later, Christy had experienced only two tantrums the entire time and none over the previous two weeks. "I can reason with her," Claudia remarked. "The extremes are so much better. Last week her cousins spent a whole week with us, and I didn't have to intervene once. The hitting has almost disappeared. She's wanting to be held much less often. It's much easier for me to parent her. No scratching or grabbing. She'll poke fun at her baby brother, but it's not malicious. Now she's back on a regular napping schedule. She doesn't strip down anymore. Christy still loves to dance, but very sweetly and not all day. I notice that she's much more focused. We even took a forty-minute walk together. She's begun to ask me to put her on the potty to poop for the first time."

It was six months later when we heard from Claudia again concerning Christy.

"My daughter has been driving me crazy for the past six weeks. Before that I felt like we were living with a different child. So pleasant, delightful, willing to listen, not upset with her brother. Such a sweet demeanor. A joy to be around. No tantrums. Her health was fine.

"A lot of her symptoms are still improved, but things are starting to fall apart. She started preschool two weeks ago. Christy clings to me until the minute I leave. She's back to her rudeness and demands and breaks down into tears easily. The past couple of weeks she wants to be without her pants again. She's singing all day long and beginning to dance more again. The word that fits her best is 'contrary.' One minute she begs me to hold her. The next she doesn't want to be touched. She asks her dad to kiss her good night then turns away from him. She's jealous of her brother again lately and tells us, 'I want him out of the family.' I feel like pulling out my hair!"

It was evident that Christy had relapsed, so we repeated the *Tarentula*. Claudia called us three weeks later with great enthusiasm. "I've seen the most amazing, radical changes. The morning after she took the last dose, she woke up a different child." Christy has continued to be a happy camper, and so is her mom. Another dose of the medicine was needed following a family visit to Israel during which Christy's patience was overtaxed.

"She's Always in My Space!"

This next story points out that even children who are very similar can need different homeopathic medicines. Hannah, like Christy, had a temper, a mind of her own, and a mom, Pam, who had also benefited from homeopathy. Pam had suffered from endometriosis and had tried unsuccessfully to have a baby for three years prior to beginning treatment with us. Within several months of taking her first homeopathic medicine, she got pregnant, and that is how Hannah's life began.

Pam first brought Hannah in for homeopathy for ear infections when she was fifteen months old. She benefited from *Pulsatilla* and *Calcarea phosphorica*. Her behavior reached a crescendo at four and a half. She melted into puddles of tears if she felt misunderstood. The fits were more major if she became frustrated or impatient. Pam likened her to an alcoholic whose temper flares at the drop of a hat. Her face turned cherry red, and her voice became very loud. Meanwhile, we noticed that Hannah began to contradict whatever her mom told us about her.

"She's sensitive to anything that might hurt her feelings in any little way," Pam explained. "What an orchestrator and organizer! Very demanding. She wants everything she sees advertised on television. Totally me first. Hannah needs me to sit with her, and she has to be touching me. Rarely is she satisfied playing by herself. She'll never ever admit that she's wrong about anything. The word that fits Hannah is 'hard.'

"If I give my attention to anyone else, she can't stand it. It makes her extremely jealous. She'll try to pull me away and be right in my face. It reminds me of how I used to get premenstrually except that she has it all the time! She convinced us to get a kitten, but she can't tolerate our attending to the kitty instead of to her. Hannah likes the kitty, but he scratches her because she plays a little too rough with him."

The previous few months, Hannah insisted that Pam deliver her directly to the teacher rather than just dropping her off at the entrance of her school. She had a reputation for being bossy with the other kids and was not willing to share her toys. There was no doubt that Hannah was very bright, but her teacher commented that her brain worked faster than her vocabulary. Quite an active child, Hannah had one more habit that annoyed her mother no end: she talked nonstop, repeating, and interrupting incessantly. Pam felt as if she had lost all of her personal space. Hannah's demanding, touching, interrupting, and chattering were just too much for her to handle.

The first medicine that enters a homeopath's mind for loquacious, jealous, self-centered children is *Lachesis* (bushmaster snake). Kids needing this medicine love to be the center of attention and will often do whatever it takes to get there. It is essential that they be first and best and most in whatever they do. The addition of a new member of the family, even a pet, can exacerbate this state by drawing attention away from the child. Because Hannah manifested all of these features, we prescribed *Lachesis* for her.

Pam brought Hannah back to our office six weeks later and was pleased to report that she was better: not as talkative, demanding, hard, or loud. Hannah leveled out even more after she was given a stronger dose of the *Lachesis*. Pam felt that Hannah was less in her face, able to play more by herself, not as tantrummy, and fine about letting her mom leave her at school. She has needed six doses of the medicine over the past two years. It has helped not only with her behavior but also with her infrequent, acute, left-sided sore throats. As we are writing this book, Hannah's expecting a baby brother to arrive in a month, and her demands have escalated, so we again repeated the *Lachesis.* She may well need another dose after her baby brother becomes the new center of attention.

Mischievous Molly

Many of us have the picture of little girls as "sugar and spice and everything nice." We have seen many who are more along the lines of "sticks and stones may break my bones but names will never hurt me"–tough little cookies like Molly.

Molly's parents bugged her. She found them just plain annoying. "They just talk, talk, talk," she complained. "And they make me do things I shouldn't have to. My teacher annoys me, too." So did her friends. And her brother. Molly showed her irritation by screaming, slamming doors, and throwing her stuffed animals around her room. Molly got a charge out of sneaking up behind people and scaring them. Her parents wanted help with her frequent blowups in which she would became out of control. Now nine years old, she had never outgrown her tendency to tantrum.

Molly rolled her eyes with disgust when one of her friends was mean to her or when her hair wasn't just right. This little girl had perfected the art of glaring. "Defiant rudeness" was how her parents put it. Nastiness. She just didn't cut others any slack. Frustration came with little provocation. She often lamented, "I hate my life and everything in it!" Her pride and stubbornness made her unwilling to admit when she made a mistake. Molly had a habit of judging others harshly, even on short acquaintance.

A talented gymnast, Molly was a natural performer and boasted that she was the best of all the kids at her gym. She loved being in motion and was at her best in front of others. Her ankles and thighs often hurt during her workouts. She had injured her foot the previous year. Sore throats at bedtime and headaches also bothered Molly. She had the habit of walking in her sleep, too.

A big fan of pepperoni pizza, Molly also loved fruit and candy. Very afraid of "big, fat, ferocious dogs" and bees, she was also frightened of riding on mountain roads and of being alone. She very much disliked hiking or walking on trails. Molly was particularly sensitive to changes in temperature.

The combination of overall discontentment and complaining, temper tantrums, obstinacy, Molly's athletic abilities, and her ankle and thigh pain led us to prescribe *Calcarea phosphorica* (calcium phosphate). Another characteristic common to those needing this medicine, which might be expected to arise a bit later in Molly, is growing pains. The desire for smoked meat, such as pepperoni, is a classic symptom of those needing this medicine.

At her first follow-up visit seven weeks later, some improvement was evident. Her behavior was worse for one day after taking the *Calcarea phosphorica,* then the anger and frustration diminished. She was more able to control her moods. Molly had more energy at her gymnastics workouts. Four months after beginning treatment, her father informed us of more changes. "Molly has responded well. There are still occasional angry periods, but the amazing tantrums have not come back. She agrees that the medicine has helped. The sore throats still bother her and she has infrequent headaches, although she complains less about her ankles, thighs, and feet."

It has been two years since we first saw Molly. Her headaches and sore throats are no longer a problem. But her parents are most grateful that her behavior has improved so dramatically—no more tantrums, no longer a pain to be around. Molly's just a nice kid.

14

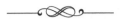

ADHD Plus Anger
Defiant Kids with Attention Deficit/Hyperactivity Disorder

As we emphasized in one of our previous books, *Ritalin-Free Kids*, ADHD is an epidemic in the United States and promises to be in other countries as well.

Children's use of Ritalin has tripled in the last five to six years, and that of newer antidepressants such as Prozac has tripled in the last three to four years, according to Peter Jensen, associate director for child and adolescent research at the National Institute for Mental Health. In 1996, U.S. physicians wrote 735,000 prescriptions for Prozac and other selective serotonin reuptake inhibitors to treat depression in children ages 6 to 18. About 1.5 million children ages 5 to 18, 2.8 percent of school-age children, take Ritalin for ADHD symptoms.[1]

There is often an overlap between children who are distractible, impulsive, and restless (with the diagnosis ADHD) and those who are defiant, angry, and aggressive. Since ADHD and conduct disorder occur together in 30 to 50 percent of cases, it is common to find aggression as a chief clinical complaint in children presenting for psychiatric evaluation with underlying ADHD.[2] In one study, of the 128 ADHD children seen at both the baseline and four-year follow-up, two-thirds also had oppositional-defiant disorder and nearly a quarter also had conduct disorder. Of those with oppositional-defiant disorder without ADHD, approximately one-third fit the criteria for conduct disorder. The authors concluded that some children with oppositional-defiant disorder associated with ADHD go on to develop conduct disorder and some do not.[3]

Having seen over fifteen hundred children with ADHD and other behavioral and learning problems in our practice, we find that some of these kids only have problems with attention and hyperactivity. Many, however, can be excessively defiant, disruptive, and disobedient. Again, for the homeopath, what is important is the degree of excessiveness and how it manifests in the particular child.

"He Slams, He Swears, and He Blames"

When you take an intense, on-the-go kid and you add defiance and aggressiveness to the mixture, you can have one big handful of explosive energy. So was the case with try-as-hard-as-you-can-to-cause-trouble Trevor.

Trevor simply didn't know when to stop. Whether it was slamming doors, pounding his feet on the wall, or finding some excuse for why he was never responsible for anything he did wrong, Trevor couldn't make himself sit still except when he was absorbed in Nintendo or playing cowboys and Indians, army, or Civil War games. He also busied himself with riding his bike, roller blading, and playing baseball and soccer.

Trevor's parents described him as "a smart mouth," especially when his father attempted to discipline him. Defensive when reprimanded, he buried hurt feelings beneath his anger. Defiance was Trevor's immediate response to being asked to do anything around the house. This youngster had a history of belligerence in the past and had been known to be destructive on numerous occasions. When he was very, very upset, Trevor declared that he hated everybody and wished he were dead. Though frequently ornery, he could be sweet when he wanted something. He had little if any patience.

Math was fun, but Trevor's verbal skills didn't come so easily. At home or school, he became easily bored. Diagnosed with mild ADHD, his parents had chosen not to give him stimulant medications.

Trevor had suffered numerous bouts of ear infections for which he received repeated prescriptions of amoxicillin. A nasal spray had been prescribed twice daily for his allergies. As a baby, Trevor was allergic to milk, similar to many infants with ear infections. He was also allergic to cats. The previous year he was diagnosed with a hydrocele (swelling in the scrotum). Trevor's dad also suffered from allergies and asthma. His father's brother died of a severe asthmatic episode. Cold milk and beef jerky were Trevor's favorite foods.

The medicine that we often give to feisty, defiant kids who become easily bored and have a destructive streak is *Tuberculinum* (a nosode). These children often have ear or respiratory infections at an early age, sometimes even from birth. This may later lead to asthma. Like Trevor, they love smoked foods and cold milk.

When Trevor returned six weeks later, he wasn't quite as mad at the world. Rages were less intense, and he was no longer pounding on walls or slamming doors.

His parents had given him the *Tuberculinum* four weeks before his follow-up visit. They found him to be generally more compliant.

At his next appointment, ten weeks later, Trevor's ears were no longer troubling him. His morning ritual of snorting and snuffing was also considerably improved. His teachers reported that he was not bouncing off the walls at school. His still disliked writing and reading, which continued to present a challenge. Trevor was still frequently defensive and disrespectful. We repeated the *Tuberculinum*.

After another two months, four months after beginning homeopathy, he was doing better. His grades had improved, he no longer slammed doors or pounded his feet on the walls, and he could sit still for longer periods of time. Trevor's writing had become considerably more legible.

Trevor's progress has continued steadily over the two and a half years we have seen him, at home and school. Each time his behavior has deteriorated, a repetition of the *Tuberculinum* has quickly brought him back into balance.

The Girl Who Swore, Spat, and Barked

One fascinating aspect of homeopathic prescribing is the differentiation of medicines, and children who need them, into the animal, plant, and mineral kingdoms. Kids needing medicines made from animals tend to be competitive, domineering, aggressive, and vivacious. Those needing plant medicines are generally more gentle, distractible, changeable, and lovers of nature. Lastly, youngsters needing mineral medicines are organized, like building and structure, and tend to want everything just so. You won't need more than one guess to figure out which is Janie's kingdom.

Janie, an eight-year-old redhead from Memphis diagnosed with ADHD, had tried lots of different prescription medications by the time her parents consulted us. Ritalin didn't work, Adderall made her spacey and caused nightmares, and she became overly excitable on Wellbutrin. When we first started treating Janie, she was still taking Imipramine, which was supposed to "settle her down." An expert at pushing her mother's buttons, Janie purposely slammed doors and messed up the wake-up setting on her mother's alarm clock—"lots of little things like that."

This little girl had a very strange way of acting out her anger. She gave anyone in her vicinity the finger as she uttered, "F— you!" not just occasionally, but one hundred or so times a day. Her parents figured she did it to draw attention to herself. Then, even more oddly, she immediately apologized. Janie was kicked out of a couple of day care centers because of her foul language and need for constant attention. Yet, despite her constant outpouring of profanity, she didn't like to watch violence on television, even violent cartoons. The only programs she was attracted to were *Sabrina,* about a teenage witch with magical powers, and *Magical School Bus,* a science program about a classroom of kids who shrink until they're very tiny and go on field trips through the body or out in space.

There were a number of other unusual features about Janie. Born with club feet and without growth hormone, she received injections of Protropin six days a week. Late to sit up by herself (age two) and to walk (age four), she was quite bright. Yet she suffered some kind of mental block. When faced with homework, Janie complained, "I can't do it. It's too hard. I need help." Placed in a special education class because of her behavioral problems and social inappropriateness, Janie had a habit of either pinching or shying away from her friends. Unfortunately, this behavior resulted in her having no friends at all. Janie was fascinated by maps—any kind of map—and even requested a "Thomas Guide" for Christmas rather than toys or dolls.

Janie was insistent on her mother's companionship and assistance no matter what she did—so much so that her mother described the two of them as Siamese twins. Bathing was a task Janie categorically refused to engage in on her own. Her mom had to stay just outside the door, coaxing her. Janie even banged her head on the door when her mother had to go to the bathroom.

Tornadoes terrified Janie, and, during storm season, she asked her mother every night if one was about to occur. Rain scared her, too; if it was raining, she called her mom from school to tell her to drive slowly. Janie also feared animals and had been bitten on the face by a dog at the age of three. Loud noises bothered Janie much more than the average child. She covered her ears if a loud truck rolled by and was wigged out by school fire drills, owing to the loudness of the bell. Her mother even had to provide her with earplugs when she went to a movie. She also had a habit of twisting her hair and chewing on furry clothing, such as velour. Janie's mother also complained that she had never been a good sleeper. Her main physical problem was recurrent headaches.

Shortly after we began treating Janie, her parents decided to take her off the Wellbutrin and Imipramine, at which time her symptom picture became much clearer. Prior to taking the medications, she had manifested a strange phobia of reflections of shiny objects. Now it was much more extreme. Janie avoided eating at the dinner table unless all the lights were turned off because of the reflection of light off several pictures on a nearby coffee table. Her parents noticed that all of the other pictures they had placed on their coffee table had been turned around so that they were not reflective of light.

Several other habits were more intensified without the medications. Janie swore and spit with great frequency. She spat all over the floor and at her baby-sitter. Another strange quirk was Janie's tendency to lick other people's feet and arms. Her fear of dogs was even greater, and she had started to make a weird, barking sound if her mother became upset with her. She avoided holding cats for fear they might scratch her. Also more exaggerated was her dread of taking a bath. And now, when the lights in their swimming pool were illuminated, Janie ran out screaming, fearing that she would be sucked down the drain.

You may recall this little girl's habit of feeling quite remorseful after her angry outbursts. Now she began to write letters of apology to her mom, perhaps twenty after each incident, in addition to her verbal apology. If her mother had not discouraged the excessive making up for these episodes, she surmised that the letters would be even more numerous. One last detail: Since we were certain which homeopathic medicine Janie needed, we inquired as to whether there had been any history of fascination with knives or with cutting herself or others. Her mom reported a wrestling match with a knife when she was three during which her mother was cut. There had been no more recurrences of this behavior.

Even if you are completely new to homeopathy, common sense alone will lead you to a certain theme in

Janie's case. Just think about, as we did, what was most out of proportion about Janie: undoubtedly her incessant fits of swearing coupled with her equally nonstop apologizing. Add to this her barking, spitting, and licking, her fear of dogs, dislike of cats, and history of being bitten by a dog. To make the puzzle complete, think about Janie's dread of bathing and her terror of being sucked into the swimming pool drain. What does this bring to mind? Janie's behavior mimicked that of a mad dog. Janie needed a very dilute, harmless, yet effective preparation of the saliva of a rabid dog. The name for this medicine in homeopathy is *Lyssin* or *Hydrophobinum*. Although the idea of giving a medicine like this to Janie might seem a bit shocking, it merely follows the concept of giving the hair of the dog that bit you, so to speak.

Lyssin is well known among homeopaths to offer considerable benefit to those with a remarkable fear of water, bathing, dogs, and the dark. It is common for people needing this medicine to exhibit animal-like, and particularly doglike, behaviors. Their outbursts of rage are reminiscent of a dog foaming at the mouth. Another strange characteristic of those needing *Lyssin* is the tendency to fits of anger followed by immediate remorse. What brings on a state like this in a human being? Often a dog bite, such as Janie experienced at age three. Another etiology is repeated torment or harassment.

Janie's response? Five weeks after giving her a single dose of *Lyssin*, her mother reported that the barking had diminished, as had the spitting and swearing. Now there were typically a couple of bad words in a day compared to the hundred or so before homeopathic treatment. She could sit in a room without going ballistic. The reflections were no longer as much of a concern to Janie. Her baby-sitter was impressed with the improvement in her behavior. Getting her to bathe was less of a battle. Janie's teachers had been equally amazed by her behavior at summer school, and one instructor had even remarked that she was beginning to be quite popular. The licking had diminished, as had other tendencies that her mother viewed as somewhat obsessive. She was still immature and continued to want her mother's company every second, but there was a significant improvement in Janie all around.

At her two-month follow-up telephone appointment, Janie's mother estimated that she was at least 75 percent better across the board. Her teachers continued to be amazed at the change in Janie. Not only did she now have friends at school, but she was busy with after-school play dates as well. Her sensitivity to shiny glass was considerably improved, as was the swearing. The headaches were completely resolved. Bathing was no longer a dreaded event, and Janie no longer found it necessary to draft letters of apology ad infinitum.

Janie has needed three doses of the *Lyssin*. Her parents and teachers marvel at the positive change they have seen in her. Now, a year after beginning homeopathic treatment, in addition to all of the other improvements already mentioned, her letters of apology have been replaced by love notes to her mom. She recently experienced a partial relapse, and the *Lyssin* was repeated.

The Boy Who Refused to Talk to Us

The task of the homeopath is to understand the patient in as much depth as possible. During our interview of the parents and child, we try to ask the children meaningful questions in a way that is fun and lighthearted enough that they won't feel threatened. Imagine our surprise on sitting down with David and his mom when we discovered that he had made a pact with himself prior to our meeting to maintain complete silence throughout the interview. The quality that we remember best about David is his silent determination. He kept his vow of silence, for one whole hour. We were impressed!

David, an eleven-year-old from Eugene, Oregon, was a creative young man, but transitions were tough. He threw tantrums when he got home from school and after returning from visiting his dad (his parents were divorced). Switching from one activity to another was a challenge. His mom described it as a problem with boundaries and limits. "My son was born talking," his mom continued. "He just doesn't understand when to be quiet or how far to push. The least little no sets him off. He yells, stomps his feet, slams doors."

David's main problem at school was concentration, which explained his diagnosis of ADHD. His teachers complained about his talking out of turn, rushing through his work resulting in mistakes, and showing below-average social skills. Other kids seemed to be put off by David's behavior. The problem could be partially chalked up to a gossipy group of peers, but the problem went further. When he finally was lucky enough to get invited to another kid's house, he was generally not asked back. There were six no-shows at his birthday party. Yet David had superb phone skills and could be articulate beyond his age. Girls either fell in love with David or were mean to him. He was usually oblivious as far as girls were concerned, except for his older sister, with whom he was forever in battle.

The daily tantrums were usually directed toward his mom, with whom he lived. When she tried to set limits, David threatened, "I hate you! I want to go live with Dad!" But deep down the anger erupted out of a sadness that his parents had separated. He disliked going back and forth between their houses, and although in his angry moments he demanded that he wanted to live with his father, once there he would call his mom and tell her he missed her. One minute he would be all hugs and kisses; the next he hated everything his mother did. Since he was only one and a half when his parents divorced, he was never able to remember a time when he had a mom and a dad together under one roof. He wrote poems about the sadness in his heart.

There was no doubt that David was talented. He dreamed of being an architect and could construct an elaborate structure out of paper or a refrigerator crate. Drama was another area in which he had inherent talent. It was easy for him to get in front of people and he had a beautiful speaking and singing voice. He often sang and hummed to himself and talked about doing television commercials in the future. David wrote fascinating, though rambling, stories about aliens, and he loved to collect Star Trek and Star Wars paraphernalia.

David's behavior problems began when his parents told him they were getting a divorce. He immediately went off to his room where he threw and banged his toys. It was easy to tell when David was unhappy because he'd lumber heavily around the house like an elephant.

Commitments weren't easy for David. He insisted on taking dance lessons, then quickly lost interest and complained that the other kids were mean to him. There was a busyness about David's mind that led him to start one thing before he finished the last. Absent-mindedness resulted in his wearing clothes inside out or backward. However, he was stubborn, persevering to get whatever he really wanted. For instance, if he decided that he wanted a particular toy, he got out the telephone directory and called store after store until he found it.

David also was quite worried about burglars breaking into the house at night. He loved crunchy and salty foods and had a strong thirst for ice-cold drinks. Physical problems included recurrent styes, blocked tear ducts, swollen eyelids, stomachaches, and recurrent sinusitis.

At times, challenges can be turned into opportunities. We used David's characteristic of refusing to answer or speak to us as one of his symptoms. Together with his talkativeness, determination, busyness, not wanting to be told what to do, and cravings for salt and ice, it led us to give him *Veratrum album* (white hellebore).

Over the next six weeks he had far fewer outbursts. Within twenty-four hours of taking the *Veratrum*, he experienced diarrhea and stomach pain for an hour. Both quickly resolved. The problems with boundaries had lessened, and his loquacity and fears had diminished. The temper tantrums were significantly better until he attended his father's wedding. The styes were gone. His mother remarked that she had forgotten to mention his offensive body odor but that it was gone as well. Since his dad's marriage, David seemed more depressed, so we repeated the *Veratrum*.

By the time of our next consultation, three and a half months later, David was doing better again. His grades were higher, friendships were blossoming, and temper tantrums were minimal. Ten months following our first interview, his friendships were still stronger. His mother estimated an 80 to 85 percent overall improvement. He began to have problems again nine months later, after he used some prescription medicine for scabies. His grades had plummeted, and he was suffering from stomach- and headaches. It was clear to us and David's mother that he needed another dose of the *Veratrum*. David, true to his determined nature, preferred to stick it out without the medicine, to handle it on his own. Two months later he did ask for another dose of the *Veratrum,* to which he had a very positive response.

It has been almost two and a half years since we first met David. He continues to do well in all ways and has not needed another appointment over the past nine months.

"It's Hard to Stay Asleep Because of My Scary Dreams"

We always hope that we can find a homeopathic medicine that produces a profound change in a child within a matter of months. This result is relatively straightforward with many of the kids we treat. There are other children, however, who, for one reason or another, are more of a mystery, and it takes longer to produce the degree of change we are all seeking. Since Kyle's mother had "been there, done that" with conventional medicine for her son, she was willing to give us the time we needed to help turn Kyle around. And we did.

Kyle, ten years old, was very articulate. Diagnosed with ADHD, depression, and anxiety, he was taking Dexedrine at the time of his first visit to us. "I feel a lot better when I don't take my medicine," he began, "more myself. School is hard. Nobody likes me. They say awful things and never ask to play with me. The other kids think I'm a jerk. I just try to ignore them, but I feel put down. Used.

"I talk a lot. And I draw. Especially eyeballs. I do lots of experiments, too, mostly in my room. Thinking's hard. People say I'm off in my own land. When I draw, I try to put my mind away from everything." Kyle's mother, Debbie, chimed in: "He folds little pieces of paper and tears them up in class. His teachers don't care for that. His desk is full of drawings and no work."

Many things scared Kyle, such as really dark rooms and kidnappers. He told his mom he was worried that she and his stepdad would get divorced. Though groundless, this concern kept intruding into Kyle's thoughts. "I'm afraid of snakes even though they're one of my favorite animals. All kinds of snakes, but particularly vipers because they're really fast. It started after I watched *Indiana Jones*. I have scary dreams all the time. One time I dreamt that somebody broke into a friend's house before it happened. Another dream was about a shark that bit off my legs.

"I can't stop worrying about this. I hate to open my windows because someone might steal me from my family. I just started reading about the mob. It takes me three hours to fall asleep. All these thoughts keep going through my brain—how people would react to me if we moved, if people like me or use me, how mean people are to me, if someone's going to come into my room and take me from my parents. Then it's hard to stay asleep because of my scary dreams."

Debbie had brought Kyle to us because of an article about our work in *Mothering*. She had no previous experience with homeopathy but was convinced it could help her son. "I'm desperate at this point. He's been on some type of medicine for ADHD since he was five.

Never any good results. I see him falling behind in school and in relationships with his peers. Ritalin, Dexedrine, Imipramine, Cylert, Buspar, Tenex, Clonidine—none of them have worked. He's really a sharp kid, but he's in special ed for math.

"Kyle's uncontrollable. He runs away, won't listen, and can't even behave in school. He wanders around the classroom touching and throwing things. He won't stay in his seat, doesn't listen to the teacher, and breaks into baby talk. At home Kyle runs out of the house, won't do what I ask of him, argues, and talks and interrupts constantly. Speakers at school complain that Kyle drills them, won't let them get a word in edgewise. He picks at scabs until they bleed. You can't communicate with him. When he's by himself with TV and his favorite toys, he's OK. Add anyone else and it's a recipe for disaster.

"And there's more. He's very hyperactive, can't color within the lines, scribbles instead of writing legibly, leaves his unfinished homework at school, tells us elaborate lies, steals, and, if that's not enough, recently he's started to cuss. Kyle is combative with his four-year-old brother and manhandles his baby sister. He got so mad that he took a hammer to a box in the garage and pounded it into oblivion. This child needs constant redirection.

"The other kids treat him very badly. He has a habit of remembering the really bad things that happen to him. Kyle has no patience at all. He's continually breaking his braces. Last night he ripped out a baby tooth that wasn't even ready to come out. Even though he knows they're off limits, Kyle has a habit of sneaking into the garage and playing with his father's power tools.

"I had a tough pregnancy and delivery—first toxemia, then he swallowed meconium. They kept him in the hospital for a week because of his low Apgars. Kyle cried for the first six months of his life nonstop. I'd set him up on the dryer, and we'd cry together. When I put him in a daycare at a year, I was told they couldn't handle him. He was a man in motion. Kyle had his own way of doing things, and no one could stop him. Actually he's just like his birth father in a lot of ways.

"Most of the time he cries about how miserable his life is. Complains that everyone has better things than him, that he has nothing, or that everything he has is worthless compared to what his friends have. He crashes all the time on his bike and skateboard. Sadly enough, he doesn't trust anyone." Kyle still had a problem with bedwetting and chewed his finger and toenails.

Kyle experienced recurrent dreams of levitating. "I'll be standing there and just float up," he explained. "This weird thing happens to my body. I feel peaceful and weightless. I've had the same feeling at times when I'm in a swimming pool holding on to the rope."

You might think that Debbie must be on the verge of a nervous breakdown, having to deal with all of this plus two younger children. It was extremely difficult for her, but she was a remarkably upbeat and good-humored woman. Nothing else had worked for her son, and she was convinced that homeopathy would work. She was willing to persist in treatment for as long as it took to help him.

Kyle was helped some by *Lyssin*, the substance mentioned in Janie's case, but the medicine that produced the most dramatic results in Kyle was *Lac caninum* (dog's milk). These two medicines are often considered to be complementary to each other. *Lac caninum* can be of great benefit to people who feel that others treat them like dogs. They feel of little value,

despised by those around them, and often turn into pas-
sive-aggressive victims. Kyle was well on his way to a
long life of misery, for himself and his family, before
homeopathic treatment.

Kyle has continued to respond well to the *Lac caninum*. His mother reported at his most recent visit, "The
teachers find him friendly and cheerful. He is blurting
out comments much less." Falling asleep was no longer
a problem. In fact, Kyle described his sleep as "awe-
some." His psychiatrist was also impressed with the
positive change in attitude and self-esteem. The dreams
of levitating did not return. We have also treated Kyle's
two younger siblings

Two Peas in a Pod

It is very rewarding to treat more than one member of a
family. Not only can it be very beneficial in leading us to
an effective homeopathic medicine, but it assists us in
more deeply grasping the family dynamics. We also find
that when more than one member of the family is
treated at the same time with the correct medicine,
deeper change occurs faster. Sometimes more than one
family member needs the same homeopathic medicine,
sort of like a genetic carbon copy. Although these traits
may or may not be passed on genetically, they definitely
seem to be transferred in some form. The next two children were remarkably similar to each other and were
helped considerably by the same medicine.

Matt and Kelsey were so similar that we will tell
their stories together. Parents will often let us treat one
of their children first. Then, if they are happy with the
results, they refer one or more of the other family members. So it was with this family. First we treated Matt,

aged six years, for his ADHD. Matt had an independent streak from the start. Matt began to walk, or we should say run, at nine months. On the family vacation when he was a year and a half old, he ran off to play with the other kids with no hesitation, seeming to not even notice that his parents were present. The vacation turned into two weeks of Matt's parents chasing him around the swimming pool, the restaurant, the hotel lobby. You get the picture.

When Matt was two and a half, his baby sister, Kelsey, was born. He became fiercely jealous. His parents could not even leave them in the same room. Matt grabbed his sister's toys out of her hand and grabbed her little throat. They fought like cats and dogs. Everything she had, he wanted. When Kelsey tried to cuddle with her mom, Matt forcefully pushed her away.

Matters worsened when Matt started school. The notes from the teacher began to arrive home within days. "He doesn't behave. Silly. Crawls under the table and makes the other children laugh. The class clown. Touches others. A disturbance in the classroom. Doesn't come when I call him. Screams. Says foolish things. Goofy." And so on.

At home, things were not going much better. When Matt's mom tried to have a conversation with his dad, he constantly interrupted. He sang at the top of his lungs to attract their undivided attention. His favorite expression, which he repeated over and over again, was "Boombah." Interspersed between the boombahs were numerous other comments that had nothing whatsoever to do with what was being discussed.

Another ploy that Matt readily used to make sure that all eyes were on him was to drop his pants. Exposing himself had led to an early expulsion from preschool. Matt delighted in breaking toys, especially those belonging to his sister. His mood changed on a dime. During his bad times, he stamped his feet, lay on the floor screaming his head off, rolled all over, and refused to let his parents pick him up. Matt was so wild that his bedraggled parents could find no way to calm him down.

One of Matt's favorite pastimes was to pretend he was a lion. He roared and asserted his role as King of the Jungle. Matt tossed and turned in bed and sneaked into his parents room every night. Needless to say, they never got a good night's sleep. He was frightened by storms, tornadoes, and insisted on sleeping with a night light. Dream themes included monsters and seeing spiders on the wall.

Matt's mom must have gotten her due reward because, according to *her* mother, she was just like Matt when she was little. She also wandered off without telling anyone, though she was fearless and lacked Matt's violent bent.

Just to keep Matt's mom on her toes, along came Kelsey, his partner in mischief making. We saw her for the first time seven months after we began treating Matt. She was almost as jealous of her brother as he was of her. Breaking his Lego constructions whenever he wasn't looking was one way to get back at him. Like her brother, she ran off all the time. When angry, she stomped, cried, and hit. Kelsey interrupted whenever anyone in the family tried to talk to Matt. She refused to follow directions and did just the opposite of what she was told.

Nobody could have predicted Kelsey's temperament by her nature as a baby. The little angel was totally the opposite of her brother: calm, sweet, loving. A baby made in heaven, Kelsey suddenly took a drastic turn for the worse. She began to wander off, couldn't sit still, and became wild. Like her brother, she stomped her feet on the floor and screamed, "No, I'm *not* doing it!" When her mom talked to her brother, Kelsey demanded, "Me, too!" She always wanted what her brother had and wailed when she couldn't go everywhere he did. Another way in which she secured more attention was by wetting her bed nearly every night.

At least twice a day Kelsey threw a full-blown tantrum, which continued until she wore down her mother and got her way. Fearless, she ran across streets without watching and rode her bike at light speed. Her teacher was not entirely pleased with Kelsey's behavior. She was sent to the office on various occasions for not listening. Kelsey had one more endearing habit: flinging herself on the laps of anyone who visited the house then showering them with hugs and kisses.

Traits often run in families, and such was the case with Matt and Kelsey. It is no surprise that they needed the same medicine: *Hyoscyamus.* It is indicated for children who tease, act foolishly and often seductively, and are wild and disobedient. All of these tendencies can be exacerbated when a younger sibling joins the family.

How did this dynamic duo respond to the *Hysocyamus?* When we spoke to Matt's mom six weeks after he took the medicine, he was getting along much better with his sister. She was able to leave them together while she dressed. The parent-teacher conference had also gone well. The teacher was very pleased. Matt was more willing to learn and no longer fooled around. Now he was able to raise his hand and wait for his teacher to call on him before blurting out his answer. His sleep was no longer restless. Matt was not acting like a lion anymore. "He's grown up. I can't believe how much he's changed!"

Matt has needed four doses of the *Hyoscyamus* over two years. His mother has no complaints.

Kelsey had a similar response. When we talked with her mom three months after she took the medicine, all was well. Kelsey was willing to do as her mother asked and had no problems in school. The fights with her brother had reduced dramatically and the two of them could play together by themselves nicely. Her dad was thrilled with the improvement in the two children. Kelsey relapsed three months later following a course of antibiotics for an infected fingernail. Three doses of *Hyoscyamus* have kept Kelsey on track over the past year and a half. The family moved to Africa, and we have lost touch.

"Everybody Picks on Me"

Melinda resembled a chocolate-covered marshmallow: hard on the outside and soft on the inside. The more we get to know her over the years, the more delightful a child she has become.

This child had a chip on her shoulder. A headstrong and stubborn nine-year-old from Montana, she loved to sing. Second came swimming. Practically a duck, she loved being in any water regardless of the temperature. Melinda didn't waste any time by raising her hand in the classroom, preferring instead to blurt out whatever she had to say. She just loved to talk on the telephone. Social by nature, making friends was an insurmountable task. "They all say I'm stupid, and they pick on me. And my mother doesn't even say anything to help," she whined. Understandably, Melinda's concerned mother decided to let her daughter work out her relationship issues on her own.

It was hard to know whether Melinda was listening to you. An exceptionally noisy youngster, she squirmed around all day long, and her attention was easily drawn from one thing to the next. Her mother shared with us, "Everything is fine as long as it's going her way. If not— bad news! She becomes unreasonably upset, persists in asking why she can't do what she wants, and won't drop it." Melinda was mouthy and constantly interrupted her parents. The only thing they had found that made an impact was to deprive Melinda of bread, her favorite food. That got results, at least temporarily. Melinda's tantrums began when she was two and were still going strong. At that tender young age, her stubbornness began as well. Melinda interrupted incessantly.

The feedback from teachers was that Melinda was so insistent on wanting things her way that the other kids got fed up with her selfishness and chose other playmates. She was continually marked down on getting along with others and following the rules. For a brief period of time her acting out extending to taking things from other people: candy from a grocery store, another child's lunch, a pen from her teacher's desk.

She had a hard time paying attention and was diagnosed with ADHD. Melinda was enrolled in a special program for math, spelling, and language arts. A bright child, she described herself as "out in the ozone." Anything that required attention was a challenge for Melinda. When others talked to her, she looked elsewhere and did not appear to be listening. Her inability to focus made reading difficult as well. At the time of her first visit to us she was on a low dose of Ritalin. The only noticeable difference was that she was less noisy.

Melinda was a skilled manipulator, a master of getting her way. One technique was to wear her parents down. They were busy with their other three children and only had so much energy to say, "No, you can't." Melinda just wouldn't take no for an answer. Although she loved animals, she didn't know how to be gentle with them. She tended to touch her younger brother excessively. On occasion she was mean and bossy toward him.

Despite her rather gruff demeanor, at the age of five, Melinda had become afraid of many things. Scary movies or television programs disturbed her sleep. Quite fearful of being alone, Melinda refused to let her mother out of her sight and often followed her around the house like a puppy. She was adamant about knowing her mother's exact whereabouts before she could go to sleep. Spending the night at the homes of her friends and relatives was out of the question. Many of these fears had diminished, but she still had a tendency to awaken with nightmares of monsters and ghosts.

Melinda had a recurrent tendency to huge warts. Her brother suffered from severe molluscum contagiosum, another wartlike condition, so it was clearly a family tendency. She had a previous history of eczema, ear infections, and a red rash on her buttocks that still persisted.

This child had the typical kid's food cravings: hamburgers, macaroni and cheese, French fries, and chocolate. The only common kid food she didn't mention liking was pizza, probably because she forgot about it.

The most unusual features of Melinda's case were her intensity, loudness, demanding nature, and underlying fears despite her tough facade. Although she had a tendency to be pushy with her friends, she was so afraid of rejection that she often gave in to them. What may not come across in Melinda's story is how much fun it is to see her and her mom. Despite any problems that she might have had, both have a contagious sense of humor. Melinda's appointments never fail to bring a good laugh, although there have also been tears, particularly concerning her social problems with other kids.

Medorrhinum produced no significant change in Melinda, and *Veratrum album* resulted in a partial improvement. The medicine that has helped her consistently over the past two years is *Natrum sulphuricum* (sodium sulphate). It was indicated owing to her strong reaction to insults from others, social awkwardness, overbearing nature, quick wit, and tendency to warts.

At her six-week return visit after she was given the *Natrum sulphuricum*, Melinda's mom reported many positive changes. She had begun to stand up for herself and her feelings and felt free to be honest with her friends, no longer afraid that if they left she would never find others to replace them. Melinda was happier and better able to get along with her peers. She now had three new friends. The overall feeling was one of greater security. The other kids weren't mean to her anymore, and she didn't seem to care as much about being liked. It was much easier to get along with her at home, which provided tremendous relief to her family. Her gas had decreased significantly. Mother and daughter were both pleased. So were we. These are the kind of deep changes that can take years to evolve, yet the shift occurred in a matter of weeks.

It has been two years since we first prescribed the *Natrum sulphuricum*. Melinda has needed only three doses and continues to do very well. All of the changes mentioned earlier have persisted. Melinda has blossomed musically and is a talented first violinist in her school orchestra. She still has some challenges interacting with her peers, but nothing like before we treated her. *Ruta graveolens* (rue bitterwort) helped her considerably during a brief episode of tendinitis of the right foot. She also benefited from a women's herbal formula for menstrual discomfort. Now thirteen years old, Melinda's main complaint is acne of the forehead, for which we have made naturopathic recommendations.

He Slammed, Stomped, and Sulked

You've heard of the half-empty glass syndrome: people who just can't seem to be happy with anything, always griping and complaining, moaning and groaning, tormenting everyone around them with their negativity. That was the story with John.

John, from Hartford, Connecticut, was fifteen years old by the time his mother discovered homeopathy. He had been on Ritalin since the third grade, and she was anxious to find a more natural alternative for her son. Getting along with teachers was rough for John. It didn't take much for him to become angry or to shut down his feelings entirely. John's mother used the words "hostile, aggressive, disruptive, and frustrated" to describe him. What finally led her to call us was fear of his violence toward her. During a recent outburst, he had drawn back his fist to slug his mother. "I just hate life!" John complained. "I wish I could kill myself." He claimed that he made these threats only to aggravate his mother, but she realized he had to be quite unhappy to say these things. John slammed doors, stomped, and threw whatever was in his reach. He was quite a sulker when he got upset.

Anger was not a new emotion for John. A very active baby, he had rocked constantly. He rarely expressed affection and did not like to be cuddled. Destructive tendencies became apparent by the age of two. He enjoyed crushing matchbox cars and bashing his toys. Accidents were commonplace. A fractured wrist and thumb were par for the course. John's behavior deteriorated even more after his father moved out. Teachers complained that he hid under the tables in the classroom and was generally uncooperative. Later, scuffles with his peers was the major complaint. John had a chip on his shoulder that wouldn't go away.

We found it significant that John's mom had always been high-strung and nervous, using tranquilizers to calm herself down. After her separation from her husband, she learned that he had been involved in extramarital affairs throughout the pregnancy and even when she was in the hospital giving birth to John.

John still rocked. In fact, his mother called him "the perpetual motion kid." A guitarist, he drummed his fingers constantly to keep rhythm. He preferred to stay up all night and sleep all day, and he was a bear during the first part of the morning. An adventurous sort of fellow, John jumped on his bike, skateboarded down steep ramps, and kept the throttle full tilt when he jet skied. Yet, uncharacteristic of his tough-guy attitude, he was quite afraid of the dark.

Food desires were nothing out of the ordinary: Oreos and milk, tuna, ice cream, spaghetti, and pizza. His most extreme features included the constant chip on his shoulder, quarrelsomeness, and a lifelong tendency to rock. As is the case with so many of the children we treat, John's basic character was established at a very tender age. He was difficult to satisfy, unaffectionate, and destructive from the beginning. These tendencies during infancy in addition to his exaggerated desire to rock led us to give him *Chamomilla* (chamomile). It has been the only medicine he has needed over the past twenty months, and he has needed three doses.

At his two-month follow-up phone consultation, John's mom reported that he was better able to understand what he was learning at school and to focus on his surroundings, despite the fact that they had chosen to discontinue his Ritalin. His teachers reported a 50 percent improvement in his behavior and learning. The throwing and slamming behavior was reduced. The child even removed his Legos from the closet and sorted them out, a first-time event. By John's own admission, he was "less hyper, not as wild and crazy," and "I don't get as mad about little, stupid things anymore."

Two months later, John's mom was still very pleased with the changes in her son. Much calmer, he was now able to have meaningful conversations with her. His inattentiveness in the classroom had continued to improve, as had his self-image. His mom estimated the degree of overall improvement at 80 percent. "He just seems to be blossoming. I feel like I have my son back. John's interacting more with the family and is 75 percent less argumentative. He is better able to understand what I expect of him and makes a sincere effort to comply." There had not been a single confrontation with John for two months. His tendency to sit and rock was gone. He was now making wiser choices about friends as well. Now, when angry, John retreated to his room to listen to music rather than to sulk.

Seven months after we prescribed the first dose of *Chamomilla*, John suffered a partial relapse. He became a bit defiant again, and his mother had received one complaint from a teacher about disrespectfulness. We gave John another dose of the *Chamomilla,* and he was quickly back on track.

We last spoke with John and his mother two months ago, twenty months after we first began to treat him. "It's been such a success story," she explained, "that we haven't needed to call you. Now John's just your typical teenager. No outbursts or confrontations. Our rapport is just wonderful. He's not even embarrassed to be seen with me like most teenage boys. He's maturing and learning to be more responsible. He weighs the pros and cons of each situation. Now the teachers tell me, 'You're the kind of parent we don't need to see very often.' And John is totally free of Ritalin." John's self-report: "I just don't get mad anymore or have crazy outbursts like when I was on Ritalin. It's much easier to be focused in school. Music and skateboarding are my life. And I have a girlfriend now. I'd say I'm doing just fine."

15

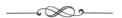

Definitely Defiant
and Disobedient
Oppositional-Defiant Disorder

Children diagnosed with ODD tend toward hot heads and fiery tempers. They hate to be told what to do—by anyone. Symptoms are usually exaggerated manifestations of child-rearing problems common to most parents. "Issues of keeping a tidy room, picking up after oneself, taking baths, not interrupting or talking back, doing homework, and practicing the piano provide adequate grist for the oppositional child's will."[1] These kids can make the pleasantries of daily life a luxury of the past. At their worst, parents are afraid to open their mouths for fear the children will jump down their throats. Any question, remark, or request can turn into a major fight. These children may continue to tantrum well into the age where they should be developing maturity and self-control. An oppositional child can push the parents, family, teachers, and everyone else in the vicinity to the limit of their patience, peace, and sanity.

Early in childhood, the child may be fussy or colicky or difficulty to quiet or soothe. The parent frequently perceives the child as difficult or "bad" and eventually anticipates unrewarding and noncompliant responses from the child. The inner experience of the child is one of helplessness, neediness, and frustration. The parent attempts to "gain control" by insisting on compliance by the child in some area of functioning, often around talking, eating, sleeping, or toileting.

Bursts of efforts at parental control and discipline with appropriate punishments and consequences are usually interspersed with hollow threats and aborted punishments. The parents frequently lose control in response to the child's continued provocations.[2]

Defiant behavior, at an early age, can be seen in both boys and girls. In a British study, interviews with parents revealed that, while fathers tended to report boys as being more aggressive, teachers and observers noted no significant gender difference, and mothers perceived girls as more aggressive than boys. Gender differences in levels of aggression become marked, in favor of boys, in the years between the third and sixth birthdays.[3]

The features of oppositional defiant disorder are described quite clearly by Dr. Jerry Weiner, editor of the Textbook of Child and Adolescent Psychiatry:

> Children with ODD frequently dawdle and procrastinate. They often "forget" or "fail to hear." A common clinical observation is that of school underachievement. They fail to do their work, forget to bring the work or assignments home, or turn them in late. Anxious parents frequently try to compensate for the child's "immaturity" or "poor organizational skills" by pressing harder, only to have the child intensify his, or her efforts . . . . In general, these children continually provoke parents, siblings, and teachers, resulting in a variety of angry,

punitive, and critical responses, during which the children argue, blame others, and lose their tempers. They often experience adaptive failure, especially at school; this, coupled with the chronic criticism they receive, often leads to low self-esteem. This is further supported by the fact that these children tend to feel unfairly picked on and feel that their behavior is reasonable and just given the unfair treatment they have received.[4]

According to other authors:

Research suggests that 20 percent of adolescents have behavioral difficulties sufficient to impair their overall psychosocial functioning, and some of these youth eventually become labeled by society as *rebellious*. Parents often become very distressed and seek counseling from their primary care physicians when their adolescents are persistently hostile, argumentative, offensive, aggressive, or hateful toward authority figures and siblings.

The most common concurrent diagnoses associated with aggressive or rebellious behavior are mental retardation; learning disabilities; moderately severe language disorders; and mental disorders, such as attention deficit hyperactivity, mood, anxiety, and personality disorders. Adolescents with major depression or dissociative identity disorder (formerly called multiple personality disorder) may exhibit behaviors that meet specific CD [conduct disorder] criteria.[5]

Oppositional-defiant children tend to demonstrate their aggression more by sneaky or covert means, in contrast to those children with conduct disorder who much more blatantly ignore or defy parental and societal rules. Defiance of authority is predominantly passive, and the violation of the rights of others is less severe.[6] Though ODD is distinct from CD, both diagnoses are considered to be predictive of adult antisocial behavior.[7]

ODD is frequently found in association with CD and ADHD. In fact, 75 percent of children with ADHD have an associated behavior disorder, generally ODD, and conduct disorder. Some children with ODD may also have psychosis, mania, or separation anxiety disorders.[8]

A Little Terror

Caroline knew what she wanted and could not be satisfied until she got it. She and her brother, Jeffrey, whose story we will mention later, were two of the most fascinating children we have ever treated.

"Caroline is a little terror" is how our telephone interview with her mother began. The family lived in New York City. Born five weeks early, her delivery was induced. She was mad from the moment she was born— such an angry face. She cried and cried until a friend gave her some homeopathic *Colocynthis* for colic.

Her mother expressed concern about Caroline's phobias to her pediatrician from the time her daughter first demonstrated compulsive tendencies. She could never take baths. In fact, she still dislikes them. Whenever she drank water, she complained of choking. Caroline was petrified of swimming. She felt very annoyed by the textures of clothes and food. Doctors were another source of terror, and she wouldn't even allow them to weigh or measure her. Another fear was cockroaches, although she loved parrots and lizards. Caroline also had an aversion to dirtying her hands.

When Caroline made up her mind, there was no changing it. One thing was sure: She wanted to do what *she* wanted to do, regardless of others' preferences. Assuming that her agenda would be respected no matter what, each day was a series of battles. Tears were commonplace. In fact, Caroline could sometimes cry all day and often woke up sobbing in the middle of the night. She loved birthday parties but insisted she was a little girl who never wanted to grow up. Another peculiar characteristic was her attraction to anything white. Chocolate, clothing, and everything else had to be white. It is not surprising that she loved marshmallows.

Caroline could be very aggressive. If mad, she hit and threw things. She put on her famous angry face that had been her trademark since birth. This child's moods changed like the weather. Her parents never knew what to expect. One moment she would fawn over her older brother, call him her Prince Charming, and affectionately blow him a kiss. The next she'd spit in his face. Caroline delighted in jumping, climbing, and hiding, especially in tight places. She had quite a problem maintaining her focus and was not one to finish what she started.

There was something else unusual about Caroline. She acted like a dog. Barking, crawling, growling, scratching, licking her parents or the floor, walking on all fours were common habits. She went through a biting stage when she was younger. Caroline also carried around her stuffed animals wherever she went. Guess what color her teddy bear and rabbit were? White, of course.

Caroline had frequent belches that smelled like rotten eggs. At the age of four to five months old, she had diarrhea on a regular basis. It still happened occasionally. The two foods that she craved the most were chocolate and fish.

Caroline is a homeopath's dream in the sense that there are so many extremely unusual features about her. We first gave her *Lyssin*. She spat, growled, scratched, barked, crawled on all fours, hid in tight places, and could be very aggressive. Kids needing this medicine often have great fear of water and rage followed by quick repentance. They can also have tremendous difficulty with sustaining concentration.

We spoke with Caroline's mother seven weeks after she took the *Lyssin*. She first experienced four days of diarrhea, a return of an old symptom that can occur briefly as part of the healing response. Then she hid even more often in tight quarters for two weeks. After that she was able to play for long periods of time, whereas before her limit of concentration was five to ten minutes. She calmed down considerably and began to act "like a normal kid." The growling and other doglike behavior stopped. Caroline was more able to play with other children. Her parents were now able to potty-train her. Her teacher reported that her behavior was excellent.

At this point she used Chapstick, which commonly interferes with homeopathic treatment, and some of her symptoms began to return. We repeated the *Lyssin* and had our next consultation six weeks later. Her attention was much improved and her attitude more flexible. If upset, now she would cry for five minutes then come back and say, "I'm happy." She no longer awakened with an angry scowl. Food textures were no longer a big issue, nor was water. However, other fears were beginning to emerge.

Two months later her father reported that she was still much calmer and softer. Anger was no longer a problem. But she had become much more clingy and fearful of strangers. Caroline insisted on looking at pictures and watching videotapes of herself as a baby. Whenever anyone referred to her as a big girl, she countered "No, I'm a baby and I don't want to grow up." She had developed fears of witches, monsters, ghosts, the dark, and animals with sharp teeth.

Generally when a particular homeopathic medicine has had a significant, positive effect on a person, we continue giving that medicine infrequently, as the need arises, over a number of years. At this point in Caroline's treatment, however, her symptoms had changed, and a different medicine was clearly indicated: *Chocolate*. For those of you chocoholics who are now conjuring up a prescription for a box of truffles, we need to tell you that this is made into a pellet form, just like any other homeopathic medicine. *Chocolate* happens to be very beneficial for people who want to remain a child and never grow up. They love cuddly animals, whether stuffed or real. There is often a tendency to animal-like behavior. They love, and often hoard, chocolate. And, like Caroline, they often have fears or disgust of cockroaches and either an aversion or liking for lizards.

Three months later, Caroline's mother exclaimed that she had seen a "97 percent improvement" overall. "She's a miracle child. Like night and day. Everything changed ten days after she took the medicine. It's so incredible. She went from naughty to nice. Now she's always saying 'Good.' Water no longer bothers her. She never wakes up crying. I was worried about her starting a new school, but she's fine. Quite easy to handle. Her father is completely amazed. I was hoping for at least a 70 percent improvement when we began. I never even dreamed of this much of a change. Her teachers and occupational therapist say she's doing great. She would never sit through church before, but now we've started going again. And you know what? She seems to have lost her taste for chocolate."

We began to treat Caroline a little over two years ago. She needed three doses of the *Lyssin*, three of the *Chocolate,* then, a few months ago, another repetition of the *Lyssin*. At one point she developed a fitful, dry cough that went away after she took *Drosera* (sundew). It is a medicine made from a carnivorous plant; that is especially fascinating in Caroline's case, since both of the other medicines that helped her have animal features. She continues to do very well.

"I'm Mean"

Medicated for "falling down seizures" since age two, Tony was behind in his classes. He wasn't yet on Ritalin, but it was just a matter of time. A seven-year-old in special education classes, Tony's teachers were putting a lot of pressure on his parents to try stimulant medication. Restless, unfocused, and aggressive, Tony got his mean streak from his dad, who had been abusive and distant toward his son. "I scream when they send me to the principal's office," Tony told us. "And I'm mean. I punch and I wrestle. But the other kids are mean to me. I hate people fighting me! And cats scratching or dogs chasing me."

At home Tony bullied his little sister, usually through hitting or tackling. Quite an active child, he loved to jump rope and play hide and seek; in fact, he practiced his jumping jacks during the interview. Tony was fascinated with lions and tigers and big cats because of their sharp teeth and ability to eat any other animal. "I like to kill birds," he boasted. His mother had actually found a dead bird in their backyard. "I want to tie everybody up so they won't be mean to me."

Living with Tony was no easy assignment. Whenever his parents asked him to do anything around the house, he stomped and called them names. He cried at the least provocation. Contrary and disobedient, Tony was forever interrupting. Mostly, he didn't listen, talked back, and threw his toys. He also picked his nose constantly. He also had a habit of grinding his teeth, and he hated being looked at.

There is an excellent homeopathic medicine for fussy, obstinate children who are extremely disobedient and may throw extreme temper tantrums up to the age of nine or ten. These kids usually pick their noses, grind their teeth, and often have a history of pinworms and seizures. The medicine is *Cina* (wormseed), and that's what we prescribed for Tony.

Two and a half months later, even Tony commented, "I'm being a little nicer." He hadn't been sent to the principal's office, was getting along much better with his sister, and had stopped picking his nose and grinding his teeth. Tony had not experienced any seizures, though he continued to take his anticonvulsant medication. A couple of weeks later, Tony's mom called to say his behavior had regressed after he had received an immunization for hepatitis B. Now his pediatrician had diagnosed him with an ear infection and was recommending antibiotics. Another dose of *Cina* rapidly cleared up Tony's ear problems, and he did not need to take the antibiotics. His behavior once again improved.

Tony has needed the *Cina* at two- to four-month intervals. Each dose has helped him considerably. Now in a regular classroom, he is interacting well with the other children. One year after beginning homeopathic treatment, Tony's EEG (electroencephalogram) was normal, indicating no seizure activity.

An Expert at Pushing the Envelope

The job description of parents is second only to that of sainthood. It is only thanks to some gene for infinite patience that they are even remotely able to cope with their really challenging kids. You will soon see that Liz was no angel. Yet her mother began our interview by calling her daughter "a wonderful child." She understood the invaluable lesson of loving her daughter no matter how frustrated she felt with her behavior. "I get glimpses of the cherub in her, but I don't think anyone else does."

Liz was so sassy that she typically wore out at least three adults in a day, to the point of utter exasperation. Baby-sitters quit as quickly as her mom hired them. This eight-year-old gave new meaning to the word *defiance*. If asked to do anything, she flared into anger or, if you were lucky, merely replied that she was too busy. Liz's nature was much like that of her father. Both of them displayed frequent outbursts of anger and procrastinated like crazy. A screamer, she would cover her ears if another family member talked to her in anything above a whisper. Liz was so noise-sensitive that movies were impossible. If in a crowd, she'd cover her ears and complain that they were ringing.

It all began when Liz was a baby. She was fine until she received her last set of polio and DPT immunizations as an infant, after which time she screamed for six hours straight. Doubled over in apparent pain, she banged her head against the wall, arched her back, and refused to be touched. The same day she developed a fever of 105 and watery diarrhea, she became limp, her face turned bright red, and she developed a glazed countenance. This turned into a bladder infection for which she received antibiotics. The crimson face and glazed eyes were reminiscent of her previous middle ear infections that had occurred after her previous immunizations. Another odd symptom that began only after the vaccinations was a tenderness and bleeding of her vulva.

Now, at eight, she still engaged in frequent clashes with her parents and grandmother. "It's her way or no way on every issue," lamented her worn-out mom. Liz's usual responses to any demand were, "Shut up. Go away" or "Get out of my life!" Although she was never physically abusive, throwing, stomping, and slamming were commonplace. Rage described Liz's response to just about anything, at least once a day—crying, yelling, and stamping her feet.

Liz's mom shared a bit of her own history. "I was probably in a huge state of fear all my life. Of everything. When I was a baby, I fell. Gazing up into my father's eyes, I saw sheer terror. At that moment I made a decision that the world was not safe. I was even scared of my mother, my brothers and sisters, of life itself. On Liz's due date my sedan was hit by another car and I suffered whiplash. I was in a state of shock."

We were not surprised to learn that Liz had her own share of fears, especially of monsters. Nightmares would awaken Liz so often that her parents had hung a "No monsters allowed!" sign on her bedroom door. The dark still made Liz nervous. Even now the monsters chased her in her dreams, and she refused to enter another room unless someone else was there with her.

There were a few other quirky characteristics about Liz. Oversensitive to just about everything, she couldn't handle noise, light, crowds, or being talked about, even if complimented. Highly prone to sunburn, Liz needed to apply an SPF 30 sunblock four to five times a day when she was outside. Indoors, however, she preferred to be totally unprotected. In fact, from the moment she came home from school, she preferred to be naked or close to it.

Add to this a propensity to be in constant motion and the teachers' complaint that she had great difficulty focusing on any one thing. "There must be something misfiring in Liz's brain," concluded her mother, who had tried every known parenting technique on her daughter.

Homeopaths always base the prescription on what is strange, rare, and peculiar about the individual, her symptoms, and her state. We always search for one thread that ties together every aspect of a person's past history and present complaint on all levels. Sure Liz was sassy and touchy, but there was much more. The intense reaction to immunizations as a baby, her equally intense reaction to the sun and to noise. The key to understanding Liz seemed to be her sensitivity on all levels—even to wearing clothing. And underlying this ultrasensitivity was the terror that she inherited from her mother and, possibly, her maternal grandfather.

The one medicine that most closely corresponds to this hypersensitivity, and that also fits particularly well her childhood tendency to high fevers with a glazed look in her eye, is *Belladonna* (nightshade). This is a case of an intense medicine being prescribed for a very intense child. Her response to the medicine was equally intense. First, her backtalking increased dramatically for three weeks, then she developed chicken pox accompanied by a fever, during which time she became disoriented. Her mother, familiar with homeopathy, had treated the chicken pox with *Rhus toxicodendron*, which rapidly relieved Liz's itching and restlessness.

Six weeks following our initial phone consultation with Liz, her mother reported that was doing quite well. The nightmares had ended, as had her sleepwalking, which she had forgotten to mention during the first appointment. Her ability to focus was better, and, consequently, her school performance was improved as well. Doodling and drawing pictures while in class had diminished. No longer as bossy, she was interacting much more positively with her friends.

Liz's mom observed a significant improvement in her daughter's self-esteem. Confidence and coordination had skyrocketed. She was getting along much better with her father. The restlessness was much less, as was her poutiness. Liz was more able to listen and be tolerant of those around her. She had not covered her ears even once since taking the *Belladonna*. The nakedness persisted, however. Her vulvar sensitivity was beginning to ease. "Liz is happier and more settled. She's even more able to joke. And to be in rooms by herself."

Another dose of the *Belladonna* was indicated two and a half months later when she had a partial relapse following her parents' divorce. When we spoke with her mother four months later, she felt that, overall, Liz was doing "fabulously." Liz now kept her clothes on, was free of tantrums, and excelled academically. Although just entering the fourth grade, she had tested at a seventh-grade reading level. "Exceptionally bright" is how the teachers described her. Far more focused, Liz could now sit down and do homework on her own. The increase in cooperation and confidence persisted. A 95 percent improvement was her mother's estimate.

"Overall, I'm delighted with the transformation in my daughter," she told us excitedly.

The only area that still needs improvement is a few fears that have surfaced. She's so afraid of needles that she won't even consider going to the dentist. Scary rides, movies, and books also drive her up the wall. She wouldn't think of picking up a *Goosebumps*. She insisted on sleeping in her mother's bed every night because her dreams frightened her so much.

Although we typically find that a child needs only one homeopathic medicine over a period of years, sometimes a subsequent medicine is indicated. In this case, Liz's new fears fit *Calcarea carbonica* (calcium carbonate), a medicine complementary to *Belladonna*. This second medicine worked very well. The needle fear subsided. She was now able to sleep alone, which her mother considered a major change. In other ways, she continued to do very well.

Liz has needed one more dose of the *Calcarea carbonica*. In the thirteen months since we began treating her, she has improved in just about every area. She's a real joy.

"I Just Can't Keep My Mouth Shut"

It is very important for a homeopath to try to understand the innermost feelings of the children we treat. Randi was another example of a girl who presented a tough exterior but was vulnerable and starving for closeness on the inside.

Randi, a sixteen-year-old teenager from Spokane, seemed like a tough cookie when we first met her. "I have ADD," she mentioned in a casual tone. "I can't learn or something. It's never bothered me. I really have no problems. My grades have varied a lot. In the past they weren't passing. I never did the work. All that mattered to me was my social life. I like to talk, about anything." Randi's mother interjected that she had been skipping a lot of classes lately. Randi went on: "I go out with friends and do whatever there is to do. We get along fine. The hardest thing for me is to stay on track. I'll start something then get distracted and move on."

Focusing was a challenge. At times the teachers barely let Randi pass their classes. A recent phone call from her teacher informed her mom that Randi was still fourteen assignments behind. "I get As and Bs at midterm, then I slack off. Then it's a struggle at the end of the trimester to catch up. My report card says that I socialize too much in class. I'm a talker. I like to talk. Just can't keep my mouth shut. I'm a loud person. If it's too quiet in a room, it annoys me."

Randi's mother filled in the details about her early years. Randi's adoptive parents had tried to have a child unsuccessfully for thirteen years. They had adopted her when she was two days old. They had no information about the birth parents, except that her mother was healthy, fourteen years old, and had at least one prior abortion. They were willing to help Randi track down her birth parents when she turned eighteen.

Trouble followed Randi from classroom to classroom. She did not follow through on completing homework. Now that she was in junior high school, she felt more free to skip class. Randi much preferred to hang out at the student center and visit with her friends. Unfortunately, she did not always make the best choice of companions. Some of her friends had gotten into trouble and into drugs. Randi had already failed one drug test. Extremely eager to please her friends, Randi copied whatever they did. Kind and loving, her self-esteem was low. In her efforts to win over her peers, she stole money or checks from her parents, then showered her friends with gifts. Some companions even convinced her to do a cash advance from her folks' bank account. Randi even lent her brand-new jacket to a friend. What she most craved was friendship.

Randi's loudness was just another attempt at gaining the attention and recognition that she craved so much. Her yell made her quite a popular member of the soccer team. Yet popularity was not always within Randi's reach. Peers made fun of her in gym class, and she responded by totally shutting them out. Compliments and positive strokes were immensely important to Randi—much more than she let on. Her parents made every effort to praise her when she deserved it. When she received an A on an assignment, they posted it on the refrigerator for all to notice.

Randi's behavior had become much more oppositional in recent months. She yelled at her father and swore at and hit her mother. When mad or frustrated, Randi fell into temper tantrums during which she threw pencils, keys, or whatever little things were around. She had a habit of retaliating against those who made her mad. If crossed, she struck back with an array of expletives. "That's how I get my anger out," Randi explained. Or she refused to talk to her friends for several days after they did something that offended her. It was very hard for her to hear her mother's feedback about her, even though her mom was gentle and loving in her manner of sharing information. Randi felt that her mother treated her "like a pig" when she talked about her faults.

On the other hand, Randi was loyal and caring, related very well to younger children and animals, and enjoyed baby-sitting. She behaved in a nurturing, motherly manner to a friend of hers who was pregnant. Randi seemed to have two very different sides to her personality: one kind and the other volatile.

Randi confided in me that even her friends told her she was mean to her mom. "We always fight. I have a bad temper, a short fuse. I can get mad over the dumbest stuff. Like when my mom won't listen to me or if I don't pass a test or if someone doesn't see my point of view. I don't like to hear no for an answer. I guess I just try to get my way as much as I can. When I get ticked off, I get loud and yell. Sometimes I have a bad attitude."

When we inquired about Randi's fears, she confessed that her arachnophobia was so bad that she'd jolt if she even saw a picture of a spider. When her friends gave her a spider in a jar, she started to cry. "It wasn't so bad until I saw the movie *Arachnophobia* four times." Randi was fond of snakes and enjoyed handling them in science class.

A junk-food junkie, Randi was at least twenty pounds overweight. Her physical complaints included recurrent ear infections, usually resulting from swimming in a pool. She had suffered profuse, occasional nosebleeds off and on since a toddler. The blood was generally bright red with stringy clots, and tended to flow from the right nostril. This had occured about ten or twenty times in her life, twice during the past few months. Randi was generally quite warm-blooded.

If we look at what is unusual about Randi, we find her to be somewhat of a paradox. Kind and retaliatory.

Loyal to a fault with her friends and insolent toward her parents. Loud and loquacious yet very sensitive to being talked about. Her terror of spiders was extreme, and even though it was prompted by a scary movie, one has to wonder why someone with a fear of spiders would submit to repeating that experience four times. Randi's nosebleeds were also excessive.

We gave Randi *Crotalus horridus* (rattlesnake) because of her striking out in anger, recurrent nosebleeds with the consistency of long, stringy clots, and extreme fear of spiders. It was only in researching this case after the fact that we discovered that the rattlesnake is the most social of all snakes. Those needing this medicine can be very talkative and irritable. Their complaints tend to be right-sided, as with Randi's nosebleeds. The only natural enemy of the rattlesnake, besides man, is the pig, which makes Randi's feeling of her mother treating her like a pig a fitting comment.

What happened to Randi? When we saw her again two months later, she had begun to read nonstop. In fact, she had started to read entire series of books. Her mother described a couple of episodes where she was much more affectionate than usual. Randi was now talking more with her parents. "I don't get so mad. Little things don't set me off as much," she told us. There were no further nosebleeds. She mentioned now that she was having daily headaches prior to beginning the homeopathy. Now they were gone.

Randi has continued to progress very well. She had a relapse following dental work, at which time she became mouthier. However, once she took another dose of the *Crotalus,* her teacher again noticed she was calmer. According to Randi's mom, the difference in her was night-and-day. "I'm thinking before I act, and I talk a lot less,"

Randi shared with us. Perhaps most important of all, she was feeling much better about herself.

At her follow-up visit eight months after we started treating her, Randi described herself as happy, calm, and relaxed. She tended to become frustrated much less often and was getting along much better with her mother. When we last saw her, Randi was enjoying her college classes, free of nosebleeds, and doing well in all areas. It has been over a year since we first saw Randi. She is doing so well in all ways that she has not needed to see us for the past eight months.

Hot-Tempered Just Like His Dad

We have heard ODD described as the terrible twos that just don't stop. That must have been how Corky's mom felt. Corky, a challenging young man from Cleveland, was either out of control or spaced out. There was no in between. Sometimes he would seem just fine all day, then, for no apparent reason, he would "go off." During those times it was impossible to reach or reason with him. Uncontrollable sobbing was accompanied by a glazed look in Corky's eyes. It almost seemed like he were having some type of seizure or attack.

Corky wasn't the only one in the family with a short temper. His dad reacted badly if things didn't go his way. Neither had an ounce of patience when events deviated from what they had in mind. Even as a baby, Corky couldn't be pacified. For the first ten weeks of his life, his mother didn't dare put him down, or he'd wail inconsolably. The only things that helped even temporarily were holding or rocking him. When he became a bit older, Corky yanked his sister's hair out in handfuls and crawled around with the air of an army commander. Not one to be held or cuddled, Corky preferred to keep moving. Constantly.

When Corky got mad, he was really mad. His mom recounted a phase of biting everyone around him without any provocation. He'd sink his teeth into his sister's shoulder, arm, or leg without a second thought. Now seven years old, he still bit or spat when he was ticked off. Corky was quite the picture of rage: curled up face, glaring eyes, and clenched fists. Then began the kicking, throwing, and striking out. Corky was not one to offer or to accept an apology.

The violent incidents had begun to mount. Recently, when his mother would not permit him to go outside, he threw a knife right over her head. On another occasion, his mother refused his demands to buy candy. Corky responded by kicking, screaming, and jumping at her, nearly pulling her over backward.

Corky was the result of an unplanned pregnancy. His parents were not getting along very well when he was conceived. He kicked so hard in utero that his mom's abdomen became sore. She contracted chicken pox when she was seven months pregnant with Corky. The main feeling of his mom during pregnancy was entrapment. Strange how children often act out the inner states of their parents. Little Corky was quite an escape artist. At the age of eight months, while his parent were attending to something else, he unlatched the screen door and crawled out into the front yard.

On top of morning sickness was the wrath of her husband, which he unleashed by calling her names and pushing her against the wall. Just before Corky's birth, his father kicked his maternal grandmother out of their house and instructed her never to return.

Mischief was Corky's middle name. Once he dragged a garden hose into the house and turned it on full force in the living room. Another time he was bent on tossing his mother's purse into a swimming pool. It was as if he took great effort to orchestrate the worst possible scenario and to act it out brilliantly.

We often find with our patients that violence is a cover-up for fear. Such was the case with Corky, who was afraid of excitable dogs, "terror stricken" about getting his hair cut, and even feared talking on the telephone. There was also an unsettling, recurring nightmare about someone drilling into Corky's skull. This dream occurred after Corky hit his head on the linoleum floor while tormenting the family dog until she snapped. His mother described his anger as unpredictable: "You never know when he's going to go off."

Corky's allergic tendency as a baby had progressed to asthma, for which he was treated with prednisone at age five. One attack followed his locking himself in the bathroom and spraying an entire bottle of perfume. Whenever he developed a cold, Corky's fever quickly shot up to 104 and his face became flushed. These febrile episodes were absolutely the only time Corky appeared calm. Food cravings included a passion for garlic cloves, lemons, and dill pickles. In fact, he could polish off an entire jar of pickles in a day.

The first medicine that we gave Corky was *Belladonna*. Usually an incorrect homeopathic medicine produces no results whatsoever, but if the medicine is very close to the correct one, there can sometimes be a temporary worsening of symptoms. Corky's behavior and asthma both worsened. At his six-week follow-up appointment, we changed the medicine to *Stramonium* (thorn apple). Very closely related to *Belladonna*, it is one of the most commonly prescribed medicines for a combination of violence and terror.

Corky has progressed very well with *Stramonium* over the past twenty months, needing seven doses in all. Within a matter of weeks he calmed down, listened and focused better, and was able to sit still. He would still throw things when upset, but the biting and spitting had stopped. Going to sleep at night was much smoother, and Corky no longer awakened at four in the morning (a detail his mom had forgotten to mention initially). He made it through a cold with no medication. Now a couple of pickles satisfied him instead of devouring the whole jar.

Four months after taking the *Stramonium*, Corky was at least 50 percent better across the board. Easier to talk to and deal with, he was now receptive to his mother's requests. Corky no longer hurt his sister daily as he had done previously. His sister was amazed that she could actually talk with Corky on a friendly basis. During his visit to his grandmother, all she could talk about was the night-and-day difference in Corky. "I even enjoy being around my grandson now," she exclaimed.

Thankfully, Corky's fears and impulsiveness decreased, and he was able to get along with other kids much better. His urge to wander was also diminished. Asthma attacks were nonexistent, even after hanging out with the family cat. Before, he pretended to cry but didn't seem to genuinely feel sad. Now Corky cried real tears at appropriate times. He was also down to just one pickle a day.

After nine months on *Stramonium*, Corky's mom estimated his turnaround at 60 to 75 percent. The steady improvement was interrupted by exposure to Pine-Sol and coffee and to a family move. Each time he reverted to some of his angry ways then did well again after the medicine was repeated. It generally took one and a half to two weeks after each dose for the positive change to be noticeable. Corky is not finished with treatment. He still needs infrequent doses of the *Stramonium*. At some point in time we expect that this will no longer be necessary.

"Nothing Pleased Her"

Positive parenting is not so easy with negative kids. Some kids seem impossible to please, no matter what. Mandy was just that sort of child and was only three years old when her parents called us for help. Night terrors were one of her parents' major concerns. Not only did she scream, thrash, and call out in her sleep, but Mandy also had great difficulty entering the world each morning. Nothing was right. Breakfast didn't suit her. Underwear bugged her. The seams on her socks were irritating. There was no way to please this little girl. When mad, Mandy let everyone know about it. She bit, kicked, hit, pinched, and pushed, never bothering to apologize.

Separation was a major trauma for Mandy. Now four, it had only been the past month that her mother was able to drop her off at day care without needing a caretaker to hold her for a while until she stopped crying. "The separation thing" prevented Mandy from going to her friends' houses to play. Leaving her mother made her nervous. Going places was fine as long as her mother was beside her.

Mandy loved it when her mother held her close. She had been an avid nurser until age two and continued nighttime nursing until three and a half. As an infant Mandy definitely didn't like water. Quite fearful of dogs as a baby, she was still cautious around canines.

Mandy's mom described her as "fiery, friendly, and animated." Inquisitive and creative, she knew exactly what she wanted to wear at all times. With her sixteen-year-old sister and two-year-old brother, she exhibited a "dominant presence." Outbursts literally flew out of this little girl. "Mandy's loud and wild. It almost seems beyond her control. The emotions simply erupt." Her threats to her brother were downright scary: "I'll chop you up in pieces. I'm gonna break your arms off." Even more chilling was the fact that she made these threats even when she wasn't angry. Bedwetting and nose picking were also problems for Mandy.

This is another child who benefited tremendously from *Stramonium*, needing six doses over the past year and a half. Within six weeks she had a much easier time separating from her mom and moving out into the world. Being left at day care was no longer an issue. Not only was she able to get herself dressed in the morning "without major breakdowns," but she tolerated a much wider variety of clothing, including socks with seams. Having decided on her own that she no longer needed diapers at night, her underwear was now dry each morning. The day care provider noted that Mandy was more flexible. Night terrors were no more, and waking in the morning was less painful. The only thing that had not yet resolved was Mandy's angry outbursts. We knew that, given the impressive response in her other symptoms, the anger should come around as well, so we gave the medicine more time to act.

In our conversation with her mom two months later, Mandy was definitely less violent. She no longer kicked, hit, or bit, although she still pinched. She seemed to thrive on extreme physical contact with people, loving to climb on them and have them swing her around. More focused, calm, and reasonable, she was better able to have dialogues with others, talking matters through to resolution. Sleep was much improved, bedwetting had come back but infrequently, and the separation anxiety was at least 50 percent better.

Four months later the bedwetting had resolved, and she was comfortable staying over at her friends' houses and being dropped off at ballet class or day care. "More affectionate, cheerful, independent, cooperative, and relaxed" were her mom's words. Her anger was much diminished, and, when Mandy did become upset, she recovered much more quickly. She had stopped pinching and bugging others. Mandy's mom estimated that she was about 60 to 65 percent better overall. Three months later her estimate was 75 percent. One more repetition of the *Stramonium* was required just a few weeks ago after Mandy's dad inadvertently let her drink some of his coffee, and her symptoms, which had been 75 to 80 percent gone, returned to a lesser degree. This is an example of why we ask our patients to avoid coffee, because such relapses are common, depending on an individual's susceptibility.

Eight Going on Eighteen

Many parents feel that kids are growing up way too fast. Exposure to sex, drugs, profanity, and the harsh realities of life come all too soon, leading some parents even to ban television in their homes or pull their kids out of the public school system and homeschool instead.

Rajani was one of those little girls who just couldn't grow up fast enough.

"Overreactive" was the word that Janice's mom used to sum up her daughter's temperament. "Rajani has tremendous problems at home. It seems as if her emotional reasoning is way off. My daughter has no understanding at all that she can't break rules. In fact, she breaks every rule in the house without any regard at all for the consequences. Time-outs don't faze her in the least."

This child, eight years old going on eighteen, had great aspirations of becoming an MTV dancer. Rajani's favorite pastime, other than, naturally, watching MTV, was spiriting away her mother's makeup, retreating to her bedroom, and dressing up like her television idols: undershirt stuffed with tissue, dangling earrings, the works. "I just can't stop myself," lamented the precocious future entertainer. "It's a sexy kind of appearance," Rajani's mother explained. "Complete with gymnastic gyrations just like the MTV dancers. Her shorts have to be rolled up just so and her dresses fitted to the nines. I'm concerned that she lacks a true feeling of herself. She'll strip off all of her clothes to look like the carbon copy of her peers. She even asks them, 'Do you want to be twins?' You'd think she were already a teenager. "

Yet Rajani, despite her seductive style of dress and gestures, was not that crazy about boys, though she did enjoy teasing them whenever the opportunity arose. However, she had no tolerance whatsoever for being teased back. In kindergarten, a boy had fallen in love with her. Rajani's response had been to give him the cold shoulder, which resulted in endless comments, often graphic, by the other boys in their class. This was so distressing to Rajani that her parents transferred her to a parochial school.

From the age of four, Rajani asserted, "I'm in charge of myself and my body . You can't tell me what to do, Mom!" Driven and stubborn, she continually complained that whatever did not go her way was unfair. There seemed to be no connection in Rajani's mind between her own actions and the consequences. Nor was she able to pick up on social cues.

Whatever caught Rajani's fancy, she did to the extreme. "When she got into cartwheels, she did them over and over and over again. I'd guess she did about five thousand of them. In the store, the house, the pool, on the ice skating rink. Everywhere! Rajani loves to spin around and run through the house. She hated so much to stop playing that we would have to drag her away kicking and screaming." A social butterfly from the time she was a baby, Rajani adored company. At eighteen months of age, she opened the front door and invited the garbage men to her birthday party. Her mother finally resorted to bolting the door.

Modesty was not one of Rajani's virtues. From the time she was tiny, she had the habit of spreading her legs wide apart and exposing her genitals. Bolting the door was manageable during toddlerhood, but now that Rajani was eight, she was too old to contain. Once when the exterior of their house was being painted, she stuffed her tight T-shirt with tissue, pulled her shoulders back, and paraded around as if she were on the cover of *Cosmopolitan*. This child loved to sing and dance and could be mesmerized for hours by watching others dance. She loved to perform dances in front of her extended family. Getting her to stop was the problem.

Despite the fact that, in some ways, Rajani acted twice her age, she was actually quite immature. She loved to make faces at her younger sister. Anything for attention. Her classmates were so annoyed by her antics that they complained to the teacher. Rajani and her sister fought like cats and dogs. The sibling rivalry began the moment the younger child was born. In fact, from the time she visited her mom and the new baby in the hospital, she lost some of her language and started to grunt. Once when her baby sister let out a piercing shriek, Rajani stuffed her fist in the infant's mouth to get her to stop. She had zero tolerance for her mother giving attention to the newborn. "You love Bindi more than me!" she wailed. Her retaliation was to try her best to get her little sister into trouble as often as possible. Whenever she passed by, Rajani set out to provoke her by pinching, hitting, or antagonizing her.

Generally healthy, Rajani suffered briefly from colic at three months and a ruptured eardrum at ten months. Fairly quiet as a baby, terrible temper tantrums erupted when she hit the first grade. The fastest child in the neighborhood, she zoomed before she walked. Accidents were a common occurrence. Still very emotional, she was "feisty" and "stubbornly independent." "During one of her meltdowns," her mom said, "I'll say 'hello' to her, and she'll snap back with 'Shut up! I had a bad day!'"

Rajani feared bugs such as red ants and mosquitoes "because they suck your blood and bite you" as well as spiders. Vampires were also scary. She loved sweets, apples, and lemons and could devour a jar of pickles in no time flat.

The first medicine that we gave to Rajani was *Tarentula hispanica*, made from the Spanish spider. The reasons for this prescription include her craving of attention, love of singing and especially dancing, seductiveness, and fear of spiders. As is generally the case with an incorrect homeopathic medicine, there was no response. We then gave her *Hyoscyamus*, indicated for teasing, seductive individuals who lack modesty and, like *Tarentula*, are motivated by their inappropriate desire for attention.

Rajani received the *Hyoscyamus* fifteen months ago and has not needed another dose. The following changes were all evident within six weeks of her taking the medicine: Her stomachaches, which her mother had forgotten to mention initially, were gone. The fighting with her sister and resistance toward her parents diminished. Cooperation was improved, and Rajani felt happier in school. She was able to recognize which outfits were appropriate for which circumstances and was flexible about changing clothes if necessary. Rajani no longer asked her mother for makeup and only polished her nails once in a while instead of religiously. The cartwheels stopped almost immediately after taking the *Hyoscyamus*. Her mother described her as "more evenkeeled." Rajani no longer felt the need to make funny faces to attract attention and began to dress for herself instead of for others. Stuffing tissue inside her shirt to mimic breasts was a thing of the past. The jealousy of her sister was considerably better. Rajani still aspires to be on television, but now as a news reporter instead of an MTV dancer.

16

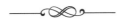

Choosing Wrong over Right
Crossing the Line to Conduct Disorder

"She was a 15-year-old doing what all teens do: trying hard to fit in." Kimberly Dotts, fed by a desire to find friends, found herself as a wannabe tagging along with the Runaway Gang, a group of kids who concocted a secret plan to leave their homes. Her parents, happy for her that she seemed to be reaching out socially, heard the excitement in her voice about her potential new buddies. The group gathered in a clearing in Shiloh, Pennsylvania, known as Gallows Harbor for a 19th-century hanging. When a distant cousin of Kimberly's worried that she might reveal their secret of running away together, one of the girls grabbed a rope, fashioned a noose, and tossed it over a branch. They pulled tight, Kimberly's body convulsed, then one girl smashed Kimberly's head with a rock to make sure she would never again be a problem to them. Seven people were right there, some standing around, some mocking Kimberly, and others helping with the lynching or hiding the body. "It was fun to hang someone," some of her friends explained. "It would be fun to do that again."[1]

Lucas Arauz, age fourteen, exhausted his options in Michigan's juvenile justice system. Lucas had a string of crimes under his belt: attempted carjacking, escape from the Berrien Country Juvenile Justice Center, an attack on his mother in the family's van during a fit of rage, two episodes of property destruction, and assault with a deadly weapon. He was diagnosed with conduct disorder, but "Lucas' mother, Erica, who succeeded in getting her son's case moved to a different county, concluded, '. . . they still don't know what's wrong with him.'"[2] This is typical of the disbelief and bewilderment of parents whose children are diagnosed with this distressing and sometimes confusing disorder.

The chief symptoms of CD, the most common psychiatric disorder in children, are aggressiveness, stealing, lying, truancy, setting fires, and running away from home. These symptoms are often associated with hyperactivity, explosiveness, impulsivity, thinking and learning problems, and poor social skills. The incidence of CD ranges from 4 to 9 percent, and it is four to five times more frequent in boys than in girls. The median age of onset in boys is seven years old, whereas in girls it is thirteen years.[3]

The rates of specific behaviors typical of CD are much higher. "One survey among youths aged 13–18 [with CD] found that 50 percent admitted to theft, 35 percent to assault, and 45 percent to property destruction; 60 percent admitted to more than one type of antisocial behavior, such as drug abuse, vandalism, and aggressiveness."[4] Another author reports that the prevalence of CD is still higher: 6 to 16 percent in males and 2 to 9 percent for females under eighteen. In a number of cases, ADHD,

Conduct Disorder: A Controversial Diagnosis?

Professionals who view CD from a developmental perspective observe the following progression of symptoms:[5]

- Young children: overt aggressive displays toward family members or at nursery school; destructiveness, aggression, refusal to comply
- Elementary school: physical aggression with peers; pushing, shoving, or fighting; conflicts with parents; stealing; lying; persistent cheating at games or in schoolwork; disruptiveness in the classroom; silent sulking versus dramatic performance; truancy; running away from home
- Adolescence: aggression, gangs, vandalism, self-aggrandizing behaviors, more aggressive assaultive or sexual behavior, alcohol and substance abuse

However, the classification of conduct disorder is a controversial and unsettled issue among mental health professionals. Depending on the constellation of symptoms, CD might include delinquent behavior, antisocial behavior, or aggressive behavior. Children with a diagnosis of conduct disorder may also be depressed, have attention deficit/hyperactivity disorder, or be psychotic. Also, the origin of conduct disorder is complex and multifactorial, with biological, psychological, and social factors having varying degrees of importance.[6] So, compared with many other psychiatric diagnoses, it is not a cut-and-dried matter.

depression, bipolar disorder, learning disorders, and psychotic disorders are also present. Current research has shown that conventional medications alone are not sufficient in the treatment of CD. These drugs may help to manage the explosiveness and rage; however, comprehensive treatment planning using psychosocial, behavioral, educational, and community interventions is necessary.[7]

The factors most consistently associated with delinquent behavior in children and adolescents are a family history of criminal and antisocial behavior, excessively harsh disciplinary methods, and family conflict. Lack of parental monitoring, regardless of the ethnic or socioeconomic group, has been correlated in several studies to delinquency and violence. The same is true of parents demonstrating low levels of warmth, affection, and support, as well as families disrupted by divorce, parental absence, and other loss.[8]

No One Successful Treatment for Conduct Disorder

One conclusion shared by all the studies on CD that we read was how difficult it is to treat. Clearly, no medications can reduce adverse family and environmental influences, which include a chaotic household and parental psychopathology; nor can social ills be treated with pharmacotherapy. In a thirty-year follow-up study, conduct disorders have been shown to have a poor outcome regarding improvement.[9]

Even the experts lament that little in the way of effective treatment has been generated for conduct disorder. This is unfortunate in light of the personal tragedy that conduct disorder can represent to children and their families and others who may be victims of aggressive and antisocial acts. From a social perspective, the absence of effective treatments is problematic as well. Conduct disorder is one of the most frequent bases of clinical referral in child and adolescent treatment services, has relatively poor long-term prognosis, and is transmitted across generations. Because children with conduct disorder often traverse multiple social services (e.g. special education, mental health, juvenile justice) the disorder is one of the most costly mental disorders in the United States.[10]

Several nondrug treatments have been identified as well established. They include parent-training programs based on behavior modification techniques as well as videotaped modeling of parent training, which teaches parents how to develop better attitudes and more self-confidence relative to raising their children.[11] Four other promising treatment approaches are cognitive problem-solving skills training, which teaches children a step-by-step approach to solve interpersonal problems using games, academic activities, and stories; parent management training; functional family therapy; and multisystemic therapy.[12]

Far too many children with conduct disorder, because they are unable to receive effective help elsewhere, end up behind bars. Robin Karr-Morse and Meredith Wiley, co-authors of the compelling book *Ghost in the Nursery*, which examines the roots of violence, cite the results of a study by the U.S. Department of Justice released in 1997.

If our present rates of incarceration continue, one out of every twenty babies born in the United States today will spend some part of their adult lives in state or federal prison. An African American male has a greater than one in four chance of going to prison in his lifetime, while a Hispanic male has a one in six chance of serving time. According to the *New York Times,* the number of individuals incarcereted in the U.S. will soon be greater than those attending colleges and universities.[13]

Aggression in the Making

Jesse was an easily overexcitable seven-year-old. A biter and a hitter, he had repeated kindergarten because his teachers did not feel he was ready to be a first-grader. Unable to keep his hands to himself, Jesse couldn't help himself from wrestling with the other boys and touching their private parts. This child had no sense of anyone else's personal space. He was just plain wound up. Teachers had to keep a careful eye on Jesse during recess for fear that he would injure the other children. He'd either punch them or peel their fingers off the monkey bars so they would tumble to the ground. Perhaps the most disturbing aspect of Jesse's behavior was that it was generally unprovoked. Jesse's mom felt a sense of urgency about getting help for her son because she was about to have a third child and feared for his safety around Jesse.

Jesse was very similar to his birth father, although his dad was no longer in Jesse's life. Both utterly disregarded others' feelings. The aggressiveness and violence also appeared to come by way of his dad. An alcoholic, he neglected his family and his business and was eventually jailed for assaulting Jesse's mother.

Also of great concern to his mother was Jesse's apparent lack of remorse or sympathy. If he hurt someone, his first response was to hide. Once, after choking another little boy, he retreated to a closet and hoped he wouldn't be found until the incident was forgotten. Jesse also enjoyed curling up in a blanket turned fortress and snuggling in his sleeping bag. Jesse's biggest fears were poisonous snakes and *Tyrannosaurus rex* dinosaurs. His only physical difficulty was a problem with visual tracking.

The medicine that best fit Jesse's case was *Androctonos* (scorpion), indicated for people with a tendency toward malicious, unfeeling behavior and unprovoked attacks of aggression. After two months, his mother reported that the calls from the teacher about Jesse fighting at school had plummeted from nearly daily to just once. He was no longer acting mean toward the other children and even did quite well at a birthday party, which would previously not have been the case. "I'm nicer," Jesse remarked.

At his next visit four months later, Jesse continued to do well. There were no more complaints about fighting or aggression. His eyes were tracking well. Jesse seemed to be getting along quite well with his baby sister. The fears of poisonous snakes and dinosaurs had evaporated, and, overall, his mother was quite relieved, especially with a new baby to occupy her attention. The *Androctonos* was given ten months ago. Jesse has improved dramatically, despite the challenge of a new sibling, and has not needed any repetitions of the medicine.

A Struggle Between Light and Dark

One of the most spine-chilling features of CD is the absence of conscience and remorse. "A thirteen-year-old boy asked a younger companion if he wanted to swing his golf club. When the younger boy grabbed the club, he found that his "friend" had heated the club with a lighter, and he received first- and second-degree burns."[14] Contrary to what some may fear, we have seen this lack of moral concern turned around with homeopathy. Christopher, a young man from Bellingham, Washington, is a case in point.

"This is a last-gap effort for us, " Christopher's mother lamented. "My son is thirteen now and has struggled his whole life. It's a lack of self-esteem. Making friends has been beyond his reach until this year, when we put him into a different school. Now he actually does have a couple of buddies for the first time in his life. He's just a shy kid. His dad and I are divorced, you know. It was especially hard when we moved here from Illinois after the divorce.

"Christopher's behavior at home has escalated recently. The violence is unpredictable. I don't even feel safe leaving him with his younger siblings for fear of what he might do to them. Adapting to change is a sticking point for Christopher. Resentment is his immediate response if plans need to be altered. Plus, he's rude. Farting, picking his nose. He thinks it's all very funny. I guess I'd describe Christopher as feeling uncomfortable in his own skin. He scratches his head and used to bite his fingernails and toenails all the way off.

"What concerns me the most is his fascination with anything violent. Weapons, guns—it doesn't matter what it is as long as it's associated with violence. And he lies.

And steals. But it's odd because he makes it so obvious, almost as if he wants you to catch him. For example, he stole another boy's Adidas jacket just because he liked it.

"Christopher is a bundle of contradictions. He can be like a saint one minute, and the next he'll slap or push his sister or say something incredibly insulting. There's the side of him that can be sweet and empathetic, loves to be held, and smothers you with hugs and kisses. Then there's the other part of him that walks in the door and yells, 'Don't touch me! Don't talk to me!' At those times he can be downright aggressive and mean. The other day he pushed me, then grabbed me by the sweatshirt. He often threatens to kill me with a gun.

"When he's bad, he swears, especially at his sister. Sometimes out loud, and at other times under his breath. It's beyond me how he can be so mean to her. How he can push and elbow her, then break her things. I got so mad at him not too long ago when he abused her that I just sat on him to break the cycle. We were in the garage at the time. I noticed him eyeing the axe by the woodpile. 'Do you really want to use that?' I challenged. He calmed down. When Christopher was only four, he clearly and premeditatedly pushed his brother down the stairs. He has a way of psychologically tormenting people. Like when he purposely switches off the television program that his sister is watching, or rips up her toys. It drives her crazy.

"Christopher once told me that he had a dark side. That he was engaged in a constant struggle between the dark and the light. He explained that there was a voice inside of him telling him to do bad things.

"Even though he desperately wants friends, he pushes away the other kids. Either he's so hyper and childish that he scares them, or he goes out of his way to please them. Not too long ago he gave away one of his favorite

CDs to another kid so he'd like him. I know that he doesn't think much of himself. He has a habit of saying, 'I'm stupid.' Even though he's bright, when he has to take a test he'll just sit there with his pencil and do nothing.

"My pregnancy with Christopher was ideal. I had a homebirth, and he got stuck. My cervix was completely dilated except for one tiny area. He came out with a cone head after I pushed for forty-five minutes. For some reason Christopher never learned to nurse as well as my other children. The preschool teacher told us he had deficits in fine- and gross-motor skills, but he made a lot of progress."

From our experience, children with low self-esteem often have a history of being criticized. We inquired if this were the case with Christopher. "His father used to tell him repeatedly that he was a rotten kid. Then he was ridiculed on a regular basis by the other children at school. That's been the case since he started school. The other kids called him 'a retard.' They tried to trip him. Once they slung him against a brick wall with such force that he broke his arm.

"We finally found the right school for Christopher. His teachers love him. It certainly wasn't like that in the past. The teachers at his other school said he was trouble. That he was disrespectful, wouldn't try, and resented being corrected."

At first Christopher wasn't very interested in talking to us. "This is so stupid," he mumbled with clenched fists. With gentle questioning, he was able to open up a bit. "The thing that's hardest for me is when I ask people for stuff and they won't give it to me. I can't seem to get over things very easily." When questioned about the conflict within him, he explained, "There's a good side that tells me to do one thing and a bad side that tells me not to."

This is another case where, untreated, the patient might have committed violent acts and ended up a criminal. One particular homeopathic medicine fit this case extremely well. The medicine is *Anacardium orientale* (marking nut) and is indicated for individuals with poor self-esteem, resulting usually from criticism (such as Christopher received from his father), torment, or abuse. They react by suffering a split within their psyches, a conflict between good and evil. If extreme, this may result in a schizophrenic break. The outer behavior is one of maliciousness, swearing, and even cruelty, usually without remorse. These children, or adults, can torment animals, which was never the case for Christopher.

After seven weeks, Christopher's mom reported, "The first week or ten days was quite a trial. Then we noticed a huge shift. For two weeks it was almost blissful. He backslid for the next two to three weeks. Lately Christopher has begun to stabilize. It's remarkable how his attitude and frame of mind have shifted. Not only is he more thoughtful and better with his sister, but he's actually willing to apologize. The one time he grabbed his sister's arm, he told her he was sorry.

"The lying has stopped, and his muttering threats under his breath is almost gone. Christopher is no longer smothering us with affection, although there are more truly tender moments. Now he cooperates and is more accepting of change. Transitions are much better. So is his focus. And, the most amazing of all, he's made a new friend and has been able to maintain the friendship for nearly two months.

"The reports from school are incredible. He's never even seen the inside of the principal's office at his new school. Last year he practically lived there.

"His grandmother called about ten days after he took the homeopathic medicine to say it was a miracle. Christopher's not scratching his scalp anymore, nor is he belching or farting. The violent talk has stopped. Even the neighbors have commented on how different he is."

Two months later the report was still very good. "All of his teachers tell us they've seen a big change. At the beginning of the school year, he was somewhat disruptive. Now there's none of that. They say Christopher is more focused on tasks, and they are very pleased with him overall. He's made some friends. They hang around together and even went snowboarding a few times.

"We now trust him with more and more responsibilities, even baby-sitting his little sister. He, in turn, is taking more responsibility for her and making sure, for example, that she puts on her seat belt in the car. It's impressive how much his confidence and self-esteem have blossomed. Even when he feels nervous off the bat, he perseveres and usually succeeds. This is the first time since Christopher was little that he smiles enough for you to see the dimples. I'd say he's about 65 percent better than when we started homeopathy."

Ten months after we began to treat Christopher, the positive change was still remarkable—75 percent better, according to his mom. At his visit, thirteen months after his first visit, she was very happy. "Just no big problems. He's cooperative, pleasant, and fun to be around. Christopher is able to handle difficult work in school. There have been no more violent outbursts. I have no complaints."

"I'll See You behind Bars"

A very fine line can separate those children enmeshed in the mental health system from those in the juvenile justice system.[15] It's a good thing Jason's mother discovered homeopathy, or he might have ended up in jail.

Jason, twelve, was on the edge of juvenile delinquency. "My relationship with my husband and daughter are being virtually ruined by Jason," explained
Jason's mom. First diagnosed with ADHD at age eight at
the local children's hospital in Portland, Jason was
given Ritalin. At least everyone thought he was taking
Ritalin—until his mother found the capsules under the
rug two years later. He had only pretended to swallow
the pills. When the evidence was discovered, Jason was
coerced into actually taking his Ritalin. He developed "a
stark look on his face and turned into somebody who
wasn't my son."

A fidgety kid from the beginning, Jason's mom
quickly pointed out that he was very different from his
comparatively angelic sister. Jana was self-motivated,
gentle, soft-spoken, and made the honor roll. Jason was
quite the opposite. At his worst, he screamed, yelled,
denied any responsibility for anything, and had "a filthy
mouth." He regularly threatened to shoot or chop up his
mother and to kill others. On the up side, Jason could be
kind, loving, athletic, and intelligent.

"Third to fifth grade was a nightmare," grumbled
his obviously frustrated mother. "The school called me
constantly to say he was mouthing off, sassy, and refused to do what he was told." Jason was pulled out of
the fourth grade after he kicked his teacher in the shins
and, when she grabbed him, jumped on her back. He
thought nothing of ripping off the blinds in his classroom. Authority made no impact at all on Jason. Defiant
with his parents, teachers, even the school principal, he
was convinced that adults were born to be challenged.
Mouthing off disrespectfully, he taunted, "I don't care
what you say." Getting Jason to do even the least thing
was a major event, whether it was brushing his teeth or
taking a pill.

"Jason drives me nuts," lamented his mom. "Fidgeting, tapping, touching, talking. He's exhausting! His sister became so fed up with him that she installed a lock on her door. Even so he's kicked a few doors off their hinges. One time he came straight at me and kicked me in the leg. I made the mistake of knocking him back and then he really came back at me. No way I'd ever touch him anymore. Spanking only made him madder, out of control.

"I do believe he has a conscience. He doesn't immediately say he's sorry, but he will apologize two or three hours later. Jason's mood can change in a flash. He's not mean or cruel to animals, though. Jason's a star football player, a fabulous skier, and he loves to roller blade and ride dirt bikes. This kid has to be first in line, first in the car, and he's always rushing to the front. He used to knock down other kids on the playground. That's why I thought football would be good for him. He was so pushy with his friends. It would inevitably end up in a fight. He's friends with a couple of disabled kids. If anyone tries to pick on them, he'll go for it to defend them.

"I married their stepfather when Jason was two and we moved from Arkansas to Oregon. He was a Vietnam vet diagnosed with posttraumatic stress disorder. The kindest, warmest man, but just that fast he turned into the most violent guy. He abused me. Destroyed me. It took me ten years to get rid of him emotionally. That man used to hit me, punch me in the nose, and even held a knife to my throat and fired a bullet into the ceiling. When I was around him, he made me feel like I was the worst human being on the face of the earth. They eventually told me he was schizophrenic. Now he's 100 percent disabled. It's so strange that he could be loving one minute then threaten to kill me the next. I'd never know which it would be. We haven't seen him for several years.

"Jason swears a lot. So do I. After playing professional pool for ten years, I'm much more verbally aggressive than the average woman."

Jason's teachers described him as "mouthy, disruptive, and defiant." Once the school called the police to subdue Jason during a fit of anger. The officer warned him, "I'll see you behind bars in a few years." He's been written up since grade 3, and usually gets over twenty-five conduct write-ups and several suspensions a year.

When we asked Jason to help us understand his side of the story, he admitted, "I don't like to be told what to do or to take orders. When I get mad at people, I scream at them. It's because they boss me around." His mother elaborated that Jason was great with younger children and older adults but quite bossy with kids his own age. "He's usually the one running the show."

Adventurous and fiercely independent, Jason was not one to be intimidated by anyone, regardless of their gender, size, or position of authority. Jason had exceled in kung fu, and his goal was to either join the army or become a professional football player. Questioned about any similarities between Jason and his birth father, his mom affirmed, "He was never afraid of anybody. One of his favorite expressions was, 'I've shot people for less.'"

Jason scared us, like a grenade waiting to explode. The combination of his explosive temper, disregard for authority or consequences, and repeated violent threats toward his mother was alarming. The one feature that struck us most prominently about Jason was how totally fearless he was when intimidated. This led us to prescribe *Agaricus* (*Amanita muscaria*). This is a mushroom that the Siberians used to take prior to battle in order to enhance their courage, stamina, and physical prowess.

Jason's mother called five weeks later to report that he was doing quite well, with fewer episodes of mouthiness and talking back. At his appointment two months after taking the *Agaricus*, it was apparent that Jason's behavior had improved considerably. Calmer and more cooperative and in a new school, he was getting A's and B's as grades instead of his former D's and F's. Feedback from the teachers was excellent. The threats of shooting his mother had not recurred. Although Jason's conduct had definitely improved, his mother felt that he had done better initially then regressed somewhat, so we repeated the medicine.

At Jason's next visit two months later, his mother was very pleased. "We had only one big row, and that's when I had PMS. I realize now why he had partially relapsed after the first dose. I sprayed his mattress with an antibacterial product, and his behavior deteriorated shortly afterward. Now there's a 70 percent improvement overall. He's getting A's and B's, and his teachers tell me that he's a joy to work with. The swearing is less frequent, and he has not gone back to his threats to kill me. He taps and fidgets, but not nearly as much as before the homeopathy."

We next saw Jason and his mother seven months after the original dose of the *Agaricus*. He continued to do very well. No threats, no fights with other people, and minimal swearing. "I still don't like others telling me what to do, but I don't get into arguments about it like I used to. My mom and I get along better in lots of ways. I'm not as mean or bossy." Jason's mother agreed: "I was ready to commit suicide when I came here the first time. I didn't know what to do. He's concentrating so much better. Now he brushes his teeth on his own instead of my telling him ninety-five times a day. He was invited to a ropes course, and, out of ten kids, he was the only one to complete the course not once, but twice. He's great at football and is becoming a fabulous video game player. Now the teachers are very enthusiastic about Jason. They tell me that he's full of potential, and they hope to have him in their classrooms next year."

It is over a year since we last saw Jason. His mother canceled his scheduled appointment five months ago because he was doing fine. She promised to bring him back if he had further problems. We called her again two weeks ago to check on Jason's progress. His grades are all A's and B's, he has "zero fits," comes home when he says he will, and is ecstatic about his electric skateboard.

Jason's aggressive behavior did not occur in a vacuum. "Exposure to violence in the home is linked to juvenile crime. Conduct disorder and antisocial behaviour, even at the age of seven, are powerful predictors of violent behaviour toward partners in adolescence and early adult life."[16] A Punjab University study on two hundred children between the ages of six and eight revealed that as many as 80 percent of the antagonistic children admitted their parents were either aggressive or violent toward each other.[17]

Rage Running Rampant in the Family

When we took Jason's case, it was clear that some of his patterns originated from and were perpetuated and even aggravated by the family dynamics. We wondered how much healing was possible for Jason unless his mother was also treated. By the time we made this suggestion to Nancy, Jason's mom, she had been impressed with the positive changes in her son and had already intended to be treated by us herself. We share her case with you along with Jason's to trace the family origins of violent tendencies in children and to show what is possible as far as healing, even over as short a time as a year.

Nancy confided, "Until I was fifteen, I felt confident and had a good relationship with my folks. Then, from fifteen until thirty, I went off the track. I got wild. It started with my parents' divorce. My mom ran off with my dad's best friend. It bothered me when I was little because when my dad left the room, my mom would sit on his lap.

"During my twenties, I began to play pool professionally. I loved it. I didn't quit until I was seven months pregnant with Jason. Those years were the hardest of my life. The kids' dad was in Vietnam. He came back with posttraumatic stress disorder. He had absolutely no respect for authority. His violence toward me really messed up my confidence. The guy was killing my soul. I thought I could fix him. He took me so far down. Convinced me I was ugly. Ruined my confidence about taking care of babies. No matter how hard I tried, I couldn't break the cycle and leave him for good. I must have gone back to him at least ten times. When he was nice, he was so nice. His validation gave me my existence. I lost my identity during that time. He did such horrible things to me. Guns, knives, choking. He drank and smoked pot.

"We had two kids in two years. Then I left. Being a single parent was the most difficult thing I've ever done. I worked part-time, and we were on welfare. My children saved my life. It was for them that I pulled myself up by my bootstraps. The kids were the most important thing to me. I never put them in day care full-time.

"Then I married a nice guy ten years ago. We had our trials and tribulations. He cheated on me until a few years ago. I feel like I've been to hell and back. After we were married for a year, he had an affair with an old girl-friend. I booted him out and came close to getting a divorce. He was a cheatin', rotten, no-good liar. He really put me through it those first five years we were together. He finally figured out that I was no dummy and wasn't gonna take it anymore. Imagine that. Two husbands cheating on me. It was devastating. I had our phone bugged. That's how I caught my husband with his ex-girlfriend. One time he went over to my best friend's house and took her to a movie. It killed me. I dumped her because she backstabbed me. Now I make sure that I don't have any girlfriends. Or, if I do, that they're fat and ugly.

"At twenty I was a pioneer in my field. You just didn't see women who shot pool for a living. I became the best player out of all the guys. You wouldn't believe how great I played. It made my family proud. The guys would watch me and say, 'Did you see that?'"

"Then I had kids, and I lost my identity. I know it's what I chose. Being a mother, a wife, running the house, making sure the kids are clean and their needs are met. But you don't have somebody coming home and telling you, 'Nice job doing the laundry!' I'm not appreciated, and the pay sucks. I'm high-strung. My mind's forever going in twenty different directions. I tell it like it is. Yikkety, yakkety, nag, nag, nag. If you asked my husband, he'd say that I yak and nag too much."

Nancy slept quite well except when she experienced nightmares about her husband cheating on her. This happened often. She awakened horrified and panicked and sometimes found that she had cried in her sleep.

The main health complaint for Nancy was PMS (premenstrual syndrome) for which she previously received progesterone injections. Her anger became so intense before her periods that she had to take Xanax (an anti-anxiety drug) so she wouldn't lose control. For twelve years her PMS was so "insane" that she cried and felt horrible for two weeks out of every month. She felt tremendous relief when her periods finally arrived. Nancy was also an inveterate cigarette smoker.

It is easy to see where Jason got his temper—mostly from his biological father, but rage ran rampant in his stepfather and mother as well. One can imagine that the seeds of his behavioral problems were planted as early as conception, if not before. Treating Nancy, in our minds, held the possibility of helping both her and Jason and, hopefully, relieving some of the tension in their interactions.

Individuals with strong issues of jealousy and betrayal by their partners, and behind-the-back intrigues, often point to homeopathic medicines made from snakes. This is confirmed by Nancy's out-of-proportion premenstrual tension and irritability that was relieved right at the onset of her periods. The medicine that best fits this combination of symptoms is *Lachesis* (bushmaster snake).

When we saw Nancy ten weeks later, there was little change, but it was evident that she was drinking coffee on a daily basis, a substance that often interferes with homeopathic treatment. She agreed to stop drinking coffee, and we repeated the *Lachesis*. At her next visit, six weeks later, Nancy had few complaints. More able to focus and prioritize, she was now able to make and follow through with a daily to-do list. "I'm going with the flow, and that's not my normal character. My last period came, and it was fine. I could deal with this. Now I can put out dinners for the family and guests, and it's not a struggle like before. Things crop up, but they no longer fry me. I have to say, looking back, that everything is better." Now, eleven months after first taking the *Lachesis,* Nancy has not needed another repetition of the medicine. She canceled her last appointment because all was going well.

We have no doubt that, if mother and son continue with homeopathic treatment, both of their lives will be transformed in a lasting and meaningful way.

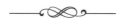

A Legacy of Abuse and Neglect
The Scars That Are Hardest to Heal

Many investigators have recognized the contribution of parental psychopathology to children with disturbed behaviors, particularly sociopathy and alcoholism, but also including more serious psychiatric disorders, such as psychosis.

> Probably the most damaging aspects of parental behavior in terms of engendering conduct disorders are family violence and physical abuse. The histories of severely behaviorally-disturbed aggressive children reveal, again and again, a pattern of physical and/or sexual abuse. Unfortunately, most of this abuse goes unrecognized and unreported, and hence rarely elicits protection from the state. In such cases, the conduct-disordered child finds himself in a potentially remediable situation: child abuse.[1]

Systematic research about child abuse may be fairly recent, but the abuse itself is unfortunately not a new phenomenon.

Most of the evidence that we have today indicates that child abuse is on the rise. If we take a broader, historical perspective, however, it would appear that there has been a marked improvement in the treatment of children over the ages. Throughout history, children worldwide have been subjected to domination, murder, abandonment, incarceration, mutilation, beatings, and forced labor.[2]

The battered child syndrome was not identified until 1962. Since that time we have come to realize that

anyone is a potential child abuser, regardless of social class or child-rearing history. With rare exceptions, the child abuser is not "sick," but troubled and isolated, as much a victim as the child. We also know more about the sociological factors implicated in the physical abuse of children. No longer do we believe that being poor "causes" child abuse. Rather, the social stresses and the scant educational, economic, and social network resources that so often accompany poverty in America are the variables that contribute to an increased likelihood of abuse. Finally, increased sophistication in our research in this area has enabled us to move beyond the idea that child abuse is necessarily transmitted from generation to generation.[3]

Family violence leaves its mark on millions of people around the world. "Several forms of violence and abuse may occur in the same family; children, parents and their partners, and older family members may be victims or perpetrators and may switch roles at different times. . . . Children in violent households are three to nine times more likely to be injured and abused, either directly or while trying to protect their parent."[4]

Sexual Abuse:
Children As Victims and Perpetrators

As recently as 1974 and 1975, when Judyth received her training as a psychiatric social worker at the University of Washington and at Harborview Medical Center, an affiliated teaching hospital, relatively little attention was paid to sexual abuse of and by children. "We were aware of neglect and abuse of children, and of the 'battered wife syndrome' experienced by some of their mothers, and we often worked hand in hand with Children's Protective Services (CPS). Part of my work was to counsel victims of rape who were brought to the emergency room by the police immediately after the assault. These victims were invariably women, sometimes in their late teens, with the exception of the occasional man, usually abused by other inmates while he was held in King County jail. Even though we were very well trained and at the cutting edge of mental health, sexual abuse involving kids rarely came up. That included incest, sexual abuse of children by neighbors and other adults or minors, and sexual abuse of children by other children. Today, of course, we are painfully aware of the far-too-frequent incidents of sexual abuse and assault involving children. It is bad enough for children to be the victims of such violence, but even as a seasoned social worker and physician, I still find it unthinkable that a child could commit a sexual crime. The times have certainly changed."

Experts agree that sexual abuse can generate an extremely wide range of symptom patterns. These patterns do commonly vary with age (for example, running away or substance abuse is more frequent among older children, and nightmares and anxiety in younger children), however there is no consistent symptom picture among sexually abused kids. Therefore, lacking a common symptom picture, conventional medical and mental health professionals can offer no one particular therapy.[5]

The sequelae of abuse in childhood and adolescence can be far-reaching. According to a 1993 report of the American Medical Association Council on Scientific Affairs:

> For those sexually abused [adolescents], consequences may include premature or increased sexual activity, increased risk of unintended pregnancy, depression, increased suicide attempts, chronic anxiety, confused sexual identity, alcohol and other drug abuse, and delinquency. For those physically abused, consequences may included generalized anxiety, depression, adjustment and behavioral ("acting out") problems, academic difficulties, sleeping problems, increased drug use, self-destructive/reckless behaviors, suicidal ideation/behavior, violence against siblings and parents, eating disorders, and aggressive behavior.[6]

Appalling though it may seem, children are now not only victims of sexual abuse but also perpetrators. Consider the following case:

> Two Florida teenagers charged with repeatedly raping their eight-year-old half-sister claim they did it after seeing a program about incest on the controversial *Jerry Springer* television talk show. The 15- and 13-year-old brothers from Hollywood, according to the police officer who conducted the interrogation, "showed absolutely no remorse. This was cold as ice. . . . There was no emotion, no cry-

ing. They never said they were sorry. It was like you were sitting at the table talking to your wife and saying 'pass the salt.'"

Springer's show has become a lightning rod for opponents of American tabloid television due to his predilection for dysfunctional guests who often engage in fist fights on camera. The *Springer* show, broadcast in 190 U.S. locations and 40 other countries, including Canada, is one of the most popular daytime television programs.[7]

Neglect:
The Suffering of the Unwanted Child

The effects of neglect on children and adolescents are not easy to pinpoint. In some cases, such neglect leads to the child being shuffled from one foster home to the next, precluding any genuine sense of belonging. This estrangement from family can lead to estrangement from society in the form of isolation, antisocial behavior, or repeated failures at establishing meaningful connections and relationships. Even in the best-case scenario, where a neglected child finds her way to a stable and loving adoptive family, the subtle, or not so subtle message of "You are not lovable. Your parents did not love you or want you" often remains deeply embedded in the psyche.

Abuse is more likely to be noticed and attended to than neglect. Often the teacher, counselor, and other educators know little, if anything, about what happens to the child or adolescent once he leaves the world of the classroom: whether someone picks him up from school or is waiting at home for his return at the end of the day;

whether he is left unattended or in the care of another child not much older than himself; whether he is adequately bathed, supervised, clothed, fed, guided, and loved. In some cases the neglect eventually becomes evident to teachers, neighbors, or others. Although Child Protective Services may be called in to address the neglect, its goal is generally to keep the child in the family, unless the circumstances are severe enough to warrant outside placement.

Abuse and neglect of adolescents may be even less noticed than that of children, in part because of the tendency among many adolescents to protect their privacy. "Although some adolescents survive abuse [and neglect] and do not seem to suffer extreme psychological and behavioral problems, many other abused [and neglected] adolescents are likely to be found in settings that reflect their response to abuse, particularly the health, social service, or juvenile justice systems.[8]

In the case of neglect, as in abuse and violence, it is easy to stereotype the drama and the characters in a cut-and-dried fashion. Obviously the victims are the good guys, or forces of light, and the perpetrators are the forces of darkness. It is easy to develop a wholehearted sympathy with the parents of a child who has been killed, raped, or injured, and to point the finger at the parents of the assailant or murderer. The same is true in the case of neglectful parents. It seems unfathomable that a parent could leave an infant unfed, unprotected, and unattended, as we read about so often in news reports. How, we may ask ourselves, can a mother, after carrying her precious infant for nine months, experiencing the pain and joy of the birth process, and then bonding with the helpless infant, even think of abandoning or ignoring her?

In many cases, however, the circumstances of the neglect are not so simple. When we delve into the personal stories of the so-called neglectful or abusive parents, or the parents of the perpetrators of the violence and crime, we soon learn that they, too, are human beings mired in suffering and pain. Often they have been the victims themselves of abuse or neglect and are simply repeating the mistakes of their parents. We all know how hard it is to shake the deeply ingrained, negative patterns that come from our parents, even with the best education and intentions and months or years of psychotherapy. These parents often lack the benefit of education, sophistication, and mental health resources. They may not, in our estimation, do an adequate job of parenting, and they may simply not know any better and be doing the best they can under tough circumstances.

Parenting can be a difficult road to follow, with all involved feeling stretched far beyond their capacities—emotionally, financially, interpersonally, and spiritually. In *The War Against Parents: What We Can Do for America's Beleaguered Moms and Dads,* Sylvia Ann Hewlett and Cornel West, after a lengthy examination of the challegnes faced by contemporary parents in the United States, propose a parent's bill of rights. This recommendation, compiled by their Task Force on Parent Empowerment, includes family-friendly workplaces, allowing adequate time for children, economic security, a pro-family electoral system and legal structure, a supportive external environment, and a climate of honor and dignity.[9]

Having diffused the blame for neglect to the society rather than just the individual parents, we can now acknowledge the high price that the many children who are the victims of neglect must pay, sometimes for the rest of their lives. The lucky kids end up in loving and nurturing adoptive homes, hopefully able to transcend their difficult beginnings. The less fortunate ones often end up profoundly unhappy and may commit acts of violence and crime.

Sidney Johnson III, executive director of Prevent Child Abuse America, confirms that child abuse and neglect are often major contributing factors to violence among adolescents and adults. Although we like to think that devastating and brutal acts of violence are unavoidable and unpredictable, that is often not the case. Most often when we look back carefully to childhood, clues suggesting possible violent behavior have been making themselves known for years.[10]

Robin Karr-Morse and Meredith Wiley, in *Ghosts in the Nursery,* warn:

> Chronic stress of neglect, which affects the development of the fetal or early infant brain; early childhood abuse and neglect, which undermine focused learning; chronic parental depression; neglect or lack of the stimulation necessary for normal brain development; early loss of primary relationships or breaks in caregiving. These are the precursors of the growing epidemic of violence now coming to light in childhood and adolescence.[11]

We have had the opportunity to treat many adopted children. We have heard many a story of an abusive husband having treated the mother of their child violently during pregnancy and of birth parents who were alcoholic, drug-addicted, and too immature, selfish, and ignorant to care for their children. In some cases the young mother makes the heart-wrenching decision to give up her child, knowing that others could provide him with a far better life than she could. However, in many cases children remain for the first few years of their lives with parents who cannot meet their own needs, much less those of their young children. Some of these kids are born with fetal alcohol syndrome or are unable to thrive; others have the strength and resilience to enjoy good physical health. But inside lie the wounds of being unloved.

His Mother Didn't Want Him

Brad, a six-year-old from New Jersey, was a kid on the go. In preschool, his teacher called him aggressive. Although he tried hard to listen and follow directions, he just wasn't able to do it, and the school recommended Ritalin when Brad was four. When his dad, Paul, declined, they were asked not to bring him back. He behaved well at his new school for a time, then started acting up again. Again, the teacher reported that he was defiant, talked back, and acted aggressively toward the other children on the playground. "He likes to do what he wants," she said. His parents gave in and started him on five milligrams of Ritalin twice a day.

Without his Ritalin, Brad put up an argument whenever he was asked to do something. "No, I don't have to" was his pat response. Then he ran out of the room, scattered his toys, and did the complete opposite of what was requested of him. When Brad became frustrated, such as when he couldn't manage to tie his shoes or get a drawing the way he wanted it, he yelled, "I hate you, Daddy" or "I'm not going to do it at all!" Flailing, throwing, and hitting followed.

By the time we first treated Brad, he was hitting the other kids on a regular basis, spitting on their food, and spitting his own food on the cafeteria floor. If his teacher asked him to complete an assignment, he threw a little tantrum. Brad had a hard time keeping his attention on what he was doing. His mind seemed to wander at every opportunity.

Brad didn't have the easiest beginning. His mother, eighteen years old at the time she became pregnant, drank and possibly smoked marijuana in the first trimester, and she smoked half a pack of cigarettes throughout the entire pregnancy. The mother, a pathological liar, had told Paul that her tubes were tied. Not true. There were apparently a number of children born out of wedlock in the mother's family. Paul and Brad's mom never married. She contemplated an abortion but didn't follow through with it. Brad's maternal grandmother, an alcoholic, kicked her pregnant daughter out of the house. She lived with Brad's father for a year, during which time a blood test confirmed that Paul was the father. Brad's mother took off, and, fortunately, Paul and his own parents adopted Brad. He still asked sometimes where his mother was and whether she were coming back. When they showed him a videotape of her at the high school prom, he asked them to replay it four or five times. The family was careful not to say anything bad about his mom.

Despite his aggressive behavior, Brad was a sweet boy. He loved animals, especially insects, pet bunnies, dogs, and dinosaurs. Though he sometimes squirmed away when cuddled by his dad or grandmother, he always wanted them around. He could be shy, at which time he talked and acted like a baby. Brad was infatuated with guns, tanks, cannons, knives, wars, and soldiers and would torment the family dog. When he recited his prayers, he gave thanks for guns. He was also fascinated by monsters, aliens, and space creatures, even though he was also terrified of them.

Brad had one favorite food, and that was chocolate. Nestle's morsels were at the top of his four food groups. He sneaked chocolate chips or chocolate ice cream first thing in the morning. Brad came by his chocolate craving honestly, though. His dad could eat half a tin of fudge at a sitting. Brad could also devour a whole jar of maraschino cherries if he had the chance.

There is a homeopathic medicine for people who have difficulty concentrating, are ambivalent about being nurtured, are wild about chocolate, and crave red-colored foods. It also is indicated when a child's mother does not want to be pregnant and can't wait until the pregnancy ends or deserts the child at a young age. The medicine is *Chocolate,* previously prescribed for Caroline. That's what we gave Brad.

The first positive report about Brad came two months after he took the *Chocolate.* His teacher remarked that he now became dizzy and felt sick when he took his usual dose of Ritalin, so it was cut in half. She was also pleasantly surprised when another child knocked over Brad's blocks, and, instead of reacting belligerently, he responded, "This isn't working. We'll just have to work it out." He was listening better and, instead of howling when told no, he was reasonable, rational, and understanding. With encouragement, he was now able to finish what he started.

There had not been a single episode of aggression. No spitting or hitting. The baby talk diminished. Brad talked more of wanting to call his birth mother. He was nicer to the dog, no longer talked about guns and knives, and, last but not least, had stopped sneaking chocolate chips.

We spoke with Brad's father and grandparents again four and a half months after he took the *Chocolate.* His Ritalin dose was still cut in half, and he did just fine on days when he didn't take any at all. Brad was able to listen, follow directions, and complete his work at school. There was still no hitting or spitting. Baby talk was infrequent, as were any references to guns, knives, or violence. He no longer threw a fit when he didn't get chocolate. They described him as a perceptive, bright, and intuitive boy.

It has been over a year since we gave Brad the single dose of *Chocolate.* He has not needed any further homeopathic treatment. His family canceled their last appointment because Brad was doing just fine. We will need to treat Brad in the future as the need arises.

A Script of Self-Sabotage

Howard, even though he and his siblings were adopted by a remarkably caring and conscientious couple, still had a hard time getting away from the influence of his earliest years. We first met Howard eleven years ago when he was only seven. His adoptive mother, Judy, brought him in after we had successfully treated her for migraines. Adopted by an extremely nurturing family at the age of four, along with his brother and sister, his future looked rosy. In fact, it promised a drastic improvement over his earlier years, prior to adoption, during which time he was abandoned at the age of one and beaten with sticks until he was black and blue. After his abandonment, Howard spent the next year or so with his father, an alcoholic, and was ultimately found wandering the streets alone. Taken into foster care at two, Howard's biological parents never even said good-bye.

At the time of his first appointment with us, at age four, his main problems were bedwetting and ear infections. At nine, it was evident that Howard was a loner, had difficulty following directions, and was unable to stay on task unless closely supervised. He had also developed headaches. *Calcarea carbonica* (calcium carbonate) helped Howard tremendously in all of these areas.

By the age of twelve, Howard had become oppositional. His social skills had not kept up with his age level, and he was unable to make friends, learned slowly, and became frustrated easily. Howard was also starting to have quite a temper, slamming doors and poking holes in walls. He began to steal and to react with defiance. This time *Baryta carbonica* (barium carbonate) benefited Howard considerably.

We didn't see Howard again for five years. Then, at the age of seventeen, he showed up with Judy in our office. "Howard asked me to bring him back so you can help him," she said. When asked how he felt about the situation, Howard replied, "I think of millions of things so it's hard to pay attention to anything. I set up my homework, then I go out and do something else instead. My grades are four A's and two F's. I feel frustrated and confused. I sexually molested my five-year-old cousin. I did it in the moment and got caught."

At this point Judy intervened, "We've discussed the options. Lots of people with criminal behavior are helped by medicines of various kinds. Howard asked to come here. I think the stealing and sexual exploration are his cry for help. School was difficult for Howard from the start, even though he's very bright."

Howard continued, "Say I'm given ten questions. Then I lay in bed and worry about it, but I don't do anything. I cover up. Give excuses. Like I'll say I did my homework but I forgot to turn it in. I like myself, but I think some of my actions are stupid. I've stolen money. I tried to cover it up, but it didn't work. The same with molesting my cousin. I put my finger inside her because I wondered what it would feel like. I'm ashamed of what I did. I steal because I like having things, and I like the risks. I usually get caught."

When we asked Howard what was most important to him, he replied, "Myself, then probably my family." He most feared getting arrested. Second came fear of dying. True to his history as a child, Howard still had trouble interacting with other people. "Some people I don't get along with at all. The things that they do and I do are completely different. I don't usually talk to them at all."

The subject of Howard's birth family came up again, partially because he had recently seen his birth mother for the first time in years. "She doesn't look very well. It seems like she's been beaten a lot. Her boyfriend used to beat her up." Judy filled us in a bit more as to his earliest years. "His biological mother ran away from home at fourteen and met Howard's father. His maternal grandfather was an alcoholic. Neither of his mother's brothers finished high school either. Howard's mother and her boyfriend married, then had Howard and another child. She was a binge drinker. It's not clear whether or not she drank during her pregnancies [which brings to mind the possibility of fetal alcohol syndrome]. His birth mom was also a habitual shoplifter. The biological father was also a drinker. He's been with the same woman for the past fifteen years."

Judy mentioned one more small detail that, to anyone but a homeopath, would probably mean nothing. It was that the birth mother and all three of her children (she had a third later by another father) had warts.

"When Howard can't have something right away, his self-sabotage system kicks in," Judy remarked. "When he stole fifty dollars at school, he was just about to be honored as the student who changed the most." Howard agreed, "I'd rather have a negative comment than none at all because it means that somebody notices me." Judy felt that the underlying theme that pervaded Howard's life was "I'm never going to make it." "He doesn't try things he knows he won't be good at. Looking cool, being noticed, covering up. Those are his patterns."

We gathered a bit more information about Howard's health history. The bedwetting had persisted until he was twelve. He suffered abdominal pain when he felt nervous, such as before tests. A couple of lipomas (fatty tumors) had been removed from his body. He loved garlic and onions.

Howard, because of the thefts and one-time sexual molestation of his cousin, was already involved in the legal system. His homeopathic treatment was one in a series of interventions in an attempt to keep him out of jail. Despite any and all help, it was really up to Howard whether he would finally allow himself to succeed in his life. Finding the right homeopathic medicine might or might not be enough to turn Howard's life around given his strong self-sabotage mechanism.

The medicine that Howard needed was now clear. A propensity for dishonesty and sexually inappropriate behavior, social isolation, covering up, warts, lipomas, and a strong craving for garlic and onions—these characteristics all pointed to *Thuja* (cedar).

Three months later Judy was happy to share that Howard was doing much better. "He's more competent and mature. The oppositional behavior is majorly decreased. Now Howard is much more able to reason. To go away, think about something, then come back and discuss it rationally. He's passing all of his classes and hasn't stolen a thing. We just met with his parole officer. Howard's been charged with child molestation, and what happens next depends mostly on him. He absolutely cannot use drugs or alcohol, cannot fail any classes or skip school, and must attend therapy. He's definitely on the right homeopathic medicine. Let's see if he lets it work."

Two months later, at his next appointment with us, Howard continued to do well and to meet all the requirements of his parole. He canceled his next follow-up, and we didn't see him again for six months. At this point Howard had been suspended from his therapy group for not completing an assignment. Judy described him as "fragile and brittle," words of special interest to homeopaths because they are specifically mentioned in the indications for *Thuja*, Howard's medicine. Judy was disappointed as she spoke: "He is able to make everyone else responsible for everything. I wonder if he needs to go to jail to really learn. We're trying hard to help him, but he's contributing 10 percent and we're doing 90 percent. He hasn't wanted to come back here. It seems like something's cooking under the surface, like he could just break apart. It's as if he's barely being held together. As if something is crying out inside of him but I don't know what." We repeated the medicine.

That was four months ago. Judy recently requested another dose. Howard is still on the edge. Homeopathy or not, the choice is his. He couldn't possibly have more encouraging, supportive people rooting for him. We found what appeared to be the correct medicine for Howard. We hope and pray that he finally chooses to succeed.

As Different as Night and Day

Carmen and Anastasia shared the same rocky start in life. Carmen was one year older. Their mother was a drug and alcohol abuser. Both the mother and maternal grandmother suffered from diabetes. The girls' mom attempted suicide several times, apparently at least once in front of the girls. Children's Protective Services tried to work with the mother for six months to keep the children in the home; however, she continued to get drunk on a regular basis. Carmen and Anastasia were subsequently removed from their mothers' home and taken into foster care by Cristina, with whom they have been since, and who had adopted the two girls. Their birth mother had supervised visitation rights for the first two years but only arranged to see the girls a total of five times. One Christmas the grandparents took the girls out for a family celebration. Six months later Carmen disclosed that one of the uncles fondled them inappropriately.

Because of the difference in their natures, the two girls have responded to their circumstances very differently. Carmen doesn't have a violent bone in her body. Quite the opposite, Anastasia has struggled with intense, violent outbursts. We tell both of their stories to illustrate the uniqueness of children even from the same family and how homeopathic treatment can help each adjust beautifully in her own way.

A Delicate Flower

Carmen was nearly three when she came to Cristina's home for foster care. Cristina brought her to see us for the first time when she was five. Beautiful and delicate looking, Carmen was quite a frightened child at first. "She was totally terrified of dogs. If she spotted a canine two blocks away, she would leap into my arms for protection. Nightmares were frequent, particularly about losing her mother or her new foster mom. Carmen's an emotionally fragile child. When upset, she cries rather than getting angry like her sister. I've had to continually reassure her to try new things and trust people." Meek and mild, Carmen even found standing up to her sister a problem, and Anastasia dominated her at every opportunity.

Carmen had a persistent difficulty separating from her birth mother, despite the troublesome circumstances of their living together. When asked what frightened her, Carmen replied, "My mom was cutting some apples and she accidentally cut her arm. Our uncle called 911. The cops took her. I cried because I thought she was gonna stay there [at the hospital] forever." This was little Carmen's attempt to make sense of her birth mother's suicide gesture. "It was scary with my mom. I'm afraid she'll die someday. I don't know if her birthday will come. I think about her a lot and it makes me cry. You know, I came out of her uterus. I'm adopted. It's scary because I can't be with my real mommy." She was also afraid of other animals and of sirens. Carmen shared one of her dreams: "I was with my mom [Cristina]. Then I threw a ball and a giant black spider came down and killed her."

Cristina confirmed that even the smallest things could bring Carmen to tears. such as when the other kids at school teased her. But mostly she cried for her mother. During these deep periods of grief, she cried so hard at times that her whole body shook. Ironically, Cristina described her as "very parentified." Her tendency to take care of those around her was so strong that she often needed to be reminded of who was the parent. Upon arriving at Cristina's, however, Carmen had regressed to needing a bottle at night. It took ten months or so before she felt bonded. Now, two years later, she still prayed for her birth mom every night.

Carmen's physical complaints were recurrent ear infections and a sensitivity of the scalp that made brushing her hair very painful. She loved hamburgers, French fries, cantaloupe, ice cream, and peanut butter and disliked mashed potatoes.

One medicine has helped Carmen consistently with all of her problems—*Pulsatilla* (windflower). She has needed three to four doses a year over the past three years. Carmen's main issue was clearly fear of abandonment. It had occurred with one mommy and she was terrified history would repeat itself. Soft-hearted and thin-skinned, this fragile flower of a child wept at the least upset.

The changes in Carmen have been dramatic: no more ear problems, considerably more strength and less tendency to cry, and lack of sensitivity of her scalp. Carmen thinks and worries much less about her birth mother and is able to assert her own will, even around her dominant sister. Her feelings are not hurt nearly as easily, even when she is teased. She is remarkably well adjusted, especially considering what she went through before being taken under Cristina's wing.

Engaging but Volatile

Anastasia, Carmen's sister, was another story and quite a handful for everyone, including her homeopath. The first things that struck us about this child was her sophistication and attractiveness. Also notable were her restlessness and volatility. Cristina took a deep breath and began, "Anastasia has always been difficult. Lots of tantrums. She used to be self-abusive. Biting herself, pulling her hair. Most of the aggression was directed toward herself. I could tell that she'd been physically abused just by observing how she treated her doll. Bedtime was horrific. She punched her doll about twenty-five times while yelling 'Shut up!' and throwing it around.

"Anastasia has never been big on impulse control. It's gotten much worse lately. Her teachers are extremely concerned. Episodes of sudden aggression without cause. One day at school she targeted another child. Anastasia followed her around spitting, kicking, and scratching her. Last week the teacher instructed her to wash her hands. Anastasia refused, then proceeded to kick and scratch the teacher. At home, when she doesn't get what she wants, she bites, kicks, and spits and becomes completely irrational and out of control. These episodes can last up to forty-five minutes. Like in the car recently when she kept scratching Carmen and pulling her hair and wouldn't stop." There was little remorse except occasionally at bedtime when she would tell Cristina, "Sorry, Mom. I had a bad day."

On the other hand, Anastasia had an engaging personality and a wonderful sense of humor. She just didn't know what to do with her anger. Bright, artistic, charismatic, and full of life, Anastasia needed frequent, if not constant, reinforcement. A leader, she had a tendency to be dominant among her peers and to tell them what, how, and when to play.

Anastasia both adored and feared animals. At times she acted like an animal herself, not only by biting and scratching but by eating only with her fingers. The use of spoons and forks were foreign to her. Her appetite was practically canine. She ate everything that was served to her. Monsters were such a nuisance that Cristina invented a ritual of sweeping them out with monster spray. Nightmares were still frequent enough that Anastasia crawled into her mom's bed most nights to escape from her bad dreams. However, despite these fears, she could also act quite brazen.

When younger, like her sister Carmen, Anastasia suffered from frequent ear infections and sinus infections. Now her only physical complaint was a tiny rash on her buttocks. Her only strong food craving was a love of bread and butter.

We tried a couple of medicines, with partial or temporary improvement for the first year: *Stramonium* and *Belladonna*. Then, because of the exaggerated and frequent temper tantrums, scratching, biting, and spitting, we changed the medicine to *Lyssin*. Anastasia was significantly better, but only transiently. Tarentula reduced her tantrums and temporarily produced an overall improvement of 90 percent. However, whatever medicine we prescribed for Anastasia wore off quickly, then, after three to six months, stopped working. This generally means the medicine is close but not exact.

18

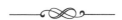

Delayed and Defiant
Kids with Developmental Challenges

The subject of childhood developmental delays associated with anger and aggression is complex. We include
in this chapter children with a variety of developmental
problems including pervasive developmental disorders
such as autism and Asperger's disorder, neuromotor deficits, and all types of developmental disabilities, to name
just a few. These conditions often overlap with physiological conditions, including head injuries and seizures.

It is reported that approximately 160,000 developmentally disabled individuals in the United States
exhibit destructive behaviors.[1] The type of disruptive
behaviors typically seen in these children include excessive aggression, impulsivity, temper outbursts, and
self-injurious behavior.[2]

Diagnosis is often difficult with these children. The
developmentally disabled represent an overmedicated
and psychiatrically underdiagnosed group. In a survey
of over fifty-five thousand developmentally disabled individuals under the age of twenty-two living in public
residential facilities, 31 percent were receiving psychiatric medications. Although this population has four to
six times the frequency of all psychiatric disorders rela-

tive to the general population, most are treated in a non-specific fashion for aggression and gross behavior disturbance.[3] In some cases, the effects of developmental disability and neuromotor deficits and abuse are cumulative. A group of Danish children, for example, were followed at birth and again at age seventeen to nineteen and twenty to twenty-two years of age. Rates of crime were found to be twice as high in those individuals having both early neuromotor deficits and unstable family environments.[4] The growing recognition that many of these children may have unrecognized anatomic, chemical, and neurological problems has led some experts to call for more participation by neurologists in the assessment and pharmacological treatment of these patients.[5]

What is most important, whether or not the diagnosis is precise, is that these children receive the help they need as early as possible from a variety of caregivers such as physicians, teachers, mental health professionals, speech therapists, and physical therapists. Early intervention can help a child or family cope with mental health problems, but it takes a commitment on the part of child care providers to keep children with behavioral problems in programs that can benefit them. Not only is it the most helpful thing to do but also a legal requirement of the Americans with Disabilities Act, which mandates inclusion of these children in classrooms by making realistic modifications in their already existing programs.[6]

According to Kimberly Hoagwood, research director for children's services at the National Institute for Mental Health, many children's problems are first noticed at school. The Individuals with Disabilities Education Act requires public schools to serve children with emotional as well as physical and learning disabilities, but there is a large gap between the 1 percent of students identified by the schools as emotionally disabled and the 4 to 8 percent estimated to have such problems. Schools, Hoagwood explains, have a disincentive to identify such students because it costs three times as much to educate a child in special education.[7]

The two cases that we have selected for this chapter are definitely children at the high end of the developmental delay spectrum. In fact, they bring into question just how close the separation is between developmental/learning problems and precocity. One can even question, in cases of children such as Gregory, which is more appropriate: a special education class or a gifted program.

Precocious and Pugnacious

Gregory, eight years old, was originally diagnosed with ADHD and pervasive developmental disorder (PDD). The diagnosis was later changed to Asperger's disorder, a high-functioning form of autism characterized by difficulties with communication and social skills and diffuse encephalopathy. By the time he was three years old, Gregory had been expelled from several day care centers. Quite precocious, Gregory had an astounding vocabulary and an excellent memory for music. In fact, he sounded like a little professor. He often invented language. He instructed his dad, "Stop that teasement." Gregory could read all day and tested at a sixth-grade reading level. His developmental kindergarten teacher was amazed at his intelligence. Tirelessly engaged, Gregory always had to be busy, whether it was talking or reading or fiddling or hunkered down in front of the computer.

When we first met Gregory in our office, the young man was quite loquacious, touched everything, was incessantly on the move, and even moved a chair to suit his play needs. His parents described him as frenetic, and they were right. Without his Amitriptyline at bedtime, Gregory was unable to sleep. He had been taking Imipramine previously but had developed such severe constipation that he was rushed to the emergency room.

Tantrums were frequent and sometimes extreme. It was as if he became locked into a particular pattern of explosiveness and simply could not calm himself. His parents had to be very careful not to set off Gregory's volatile temper. Once wound up, there was no way to interrupt the pattern. His anger just had to play itself out. Gregory's outbursts got him into frequent hot water at school. He was held in from recess for fighting with the other children, tore up lists of spelling words because they were too easy, and walked away if reprimanded. Gregory squeezed, hit, grabbed, threw dirt, and even bit his classmates. A voracious reader, he raced around his school library in a frenzy, knocking down books in his path, which prompted the librarian to request that he not return. Simply put, he was out of control. Not only did this type of behavior occur at home and at school; he was also expelled from summer camp and an after-school activity program. When we asked how he felt inside, Gregory reported a "weird feeling in his stomach as if a creature were inside gnawing on the walls."

When we inquired about what frightened Gregory, he replied, "I don't like hearing ghost stories or anything spooky or scary. They can give me a nightmare. When I go to bed, I can't get those things off my mind. Sometimes it's like being in a dark crystal with the Emperor, the Blue Wolf part of Sky Island, and Zog the Sea Monster." He feared being in the woods alone for fear that he might be kidnapped and was very careful to never leave the car door open unless his mom or dad was there because someone might grab him out of the window. Gregory insisted that his dad be with him if it were dark and on having a light on at night. His fears had escalated recently to the degree that he asked his mom to keep him company in bed.

Making friends was very tough for Gregory, in part because he had the habit of interrupting and talking out of turn. Although his bank of information and vocabulary were far beyond his chronological age, he could not sustain reciprocal conversation. Picking up on nonverbal communication or the feelings of others was beyond Gregory's grasp. He talked nonstop, regardless of whatever activity or conversation was taking place

We often hear from parents, "He ran before he walked." Gregory, a case in point, learned to walk at ten months. In no time flat, the child mastered racing around "as if King Kong had burst out of a cage." He tore around stores like a wild man, screaming whenever his desires went unsatisfied. His mom described him as overwhelming, unable to restrain himself, and maximally impulsive. When he was two, Gregory's parents, by default, parted with all of their house plants. At five, upon becoming enraged at his baby-sitter, he flipped over a full-size couch. Gregory shrieked at strangers, weeping inconsolably until they left. Yet he was at his prime when he had an opportunity to show off for new people.

This child was articulate and charming, when he wanted to be. If he didn't, however, he refused to answer and resembled a smoldering volcano. Reciting facts from his encyclopedic memory, Gregory insisted he was right about most things and called his parents names if they didn't agree with him. His memory and ability to figure things out were remarkable. At two and a half, he was capable of putting together puzzles that would baffle many a five-year-old. Though his sense of humor was charming, he tended to laugh loudly and at inappropriate moments.

From the time Gregory was an infant, he was bothered by colic. At two he had surgery for an undescended left testicle and six months later was hospitalized with severe asthma, after spending an afternoon in a home day care with four cats and a dog.

The combination of Gregory's terror of the dark and of being kidnapped, combined with his aggressiveness and sensation of something alive in his stomach, led us to prescribe *Stramonium* (thorn apple). It may seem that this medicine is overrepresented in this book, but it is one of the medicines we most commonly prescribe for children with a combination of violent behavior and underlying terror. We wonder how much of this exaggerated fear is generated by vicariously experiencing media murder after murder.

Two weeks after taking the medicine, Gregory experienced a significant improvement in the violence, according to his parents. Two months later, he continued to improve, exhibited much less violent behavior, was considerably less fearful of the dark, and was better able to respond appropriately. His parents reported, "We see the true kid—very loving, easy to please, a wonderful temperament."

Over the past two and a half years, the improvement continues in a number of areas. Gregory was moved to a mainstream classroom where he is doing very well, and his teacher is gradually adding more challenging subjects. Though still a high-maintenance child with a tendency to persevere on one chosen activity, he has progressed remarkably. He is more receptive to negotiation and talking out problems. His social skills have advanced to the point where he is able to establish friendships. Gregory reads and writes at a tenth-grade level and exhibits a definite talent in creative writing. His last teacher was so fond of him that she hated to see him leave her classroom. Gregory's neurologist has recommended that he taper off his dosage of Amitriptyline. Temper flare-ups are infrequent, usually occurring only if he stays up too late. Gregory's strong will and obstinancy continue to be a problem, but his aggressiveness has diminished considerably.

It is extremely gratifying to see the improvement in children like Gregory. This bright, engaging child was extremely limited by his excessive behaviors, flare-ups of anger, and social inappropriateness. Though Gregory still has quite a way to go, he is more able to interact appropriately with his peers and parents.

A Fascination for Blood and Gore

Jeffrey was, according to our perceptions, a child who was misunderstood by mental health professionals. They not only couldn't agree on a diagnosis or help him to any significant degree, but they had widely varying interpretations of Jeffrey's inner world.

Jeffrey, aged seven, was likeable, friendly, and charming. (We have already shared in chapter 15 the story of his sister, Caroline, whose angry outbursts abated with homeopathy.) This little boy was extremely sensitive to the least slight. As his mother described him, "You can break his heart in two seconds." He nearly collapsed when his parents suggested that he didn't do something just right. Taunting by his friends left him devastated. But what was the most out of proportion about Jeffrey was his obsession with blood, nearly his only topic of conversation. "Mommy, I imagined cutting the monster's throat. The blood's coming out!"

It all began when Jeffrey was three and a half and the kids at school bullied him for one year straight. They beat him up almost daily, which rendered him psychologically traumatized. Around the same time he became very accident-prone. One kid kicked him in the mouth, causing him to lose two front teeth, both of which were already loose. The only tactic that this gentle fellow could manufacture to defend himself was to make up scary stories. And at this he was a master. His tales were so convincing that the school complained because kids were having sleep problems after hearing them. This child also had an incredible ability to memorize poetry, but he was only interested in scary poems.

At first his parents thought this habit was humorous and entertaining. Then it got out of control. Blood, monsters, and vampires were all that Jeffrey would think and talk about. For instance: "It was dark. A boy was walking through the forest. He found an alien's house. The alien had lots of arms. Suddenly out came a big hand. Then the alien spit poison and the boy died." Jeffrey's stories always seemed to end with someone dying, or the conclusion was left unfinished.

Jeffrey had obsessive tendencies. He picked his arms until they bled and even fantasized about drinking blood and blood oozing from someone's throat. He loved Dracula and any kind of story in which there was cutting or stabbing. As he shopped with his mom at the supermarket, Jeffrey would playfully grab at her neck. At two, he picked out a vampire costume for Halloween then delighted in wearing it for months after. Jeffrey's storytelling knew no limits. While driving in the car with his mother, he would launch into one of his tales, oblivious to the fact that she had gotten out to fill the gas tank. When she eased herself back into the car, he was still talking as if she had never left.

In addition to his obsession with blood, Jeffrey was also preoccupied with germs. If someone coughed, he'd leave the room. He was a frequent hand washer and wouldn't let anyone touch his food. Toothbrushing was excessive to avoid any possibility of cavities. The word *germs* came out numerous times each day. Jeffrey was quite attached to rituals and needed his mother to repeat over and over that she loved him.

Not too surprisingly, Jeffrey experienced lots of fears. He was scared of the dark, ants, sharks, and dogs; of being grabbed by something frightening; and of being buried alive. Quite fearful of losing his mother, he ran out to protect her whenever she left the house, even though he feared being attacked himself. Jeffrey was even afraid of his own scary stories! Jeffrey awakened every night from 2 to 4 A.M. and fled to his parents' bed for protection. Reassurance came in the form of his "friends" in the attic who came down and rescued him from danger. The only problem was the family had no attic.

The strangest thing was that Jeffrey wouldn't hurt a fly, even though he could have gotten his blue belt in karate. He wouldn't even push another child. To his great disappointment, Jeffrey had only one friend at school. A psychologist described him as withdrawn, a loner, so much in his own world that he was unable to relate to the other kids. Most of the time he felt rejected and hurt. Even when talking to the other children, Jeffrey would talk to himself at the same time.

Jeffrey suffered from frequent headaches, sometimes brought on from having to make even the simplest decision. He had a history of asthma and had taken antibiotics off and on from age two to four for recurrent bronchitis and ear infections. Jeffrey seemed much more tired than you would expect from a child his age. There had been a problem with bedwetting until one month before his mother first called us.

A homeopath always asks about the mother's pregnancy, because this description often leads us to clues as to which medicine to prescribe. Jeffrey's mom suffered from depression during the first two months of her pregnancy. She became understandably anxious after her obstetrician warned her that her child might have brain damage. Labor progressed well until his heartbeat no longer registered. The idea of a Caesarean section must have been quite an incentive, because the mere mention of it caused her to push Jeffrey right out.

Jeffrey's mom described him as a perfect baby— maybe a bit too perfect because he rarely cried and was almost passive. Slow to develop, at the age of one year he still had the fine-motor skills of a three-month-old and was unable to even grab a raisin. He didn't walk until he the age of fifteen months.

Although a seven-year-old at a tenth-grade level, Jeffrey was placed in a school for learning-disabled children. His teacher described his writing as disorganized and dyslexic. When he drew pictures of people or creatures, all of the limbs came out of the head. Jeffrey's diagnoses ranged from obsessive-compulsive disorder and bipolar disorder to Asperger's disorder.

Jeffrey is one of the most fascinating children we have ever treated. So many violent thoughts in the mind of such a kind and gentle child. And so much harassment of this sweet little boy by his peers. We believe that it is to Jeffrey's credit that he invented such a creative, harmless method of surviving the incessant persecution by his peers. Many children in this situation would have manifested their violence outwardly. Jeffrey turned it within.

The medicine that has helped Jeffrey consistently and dramatically is *China officinalis* (Peruvian bark). It fits people who are timid and passive in a Caspar Milquetoast fashion and who retreat to the recesses of their mind in which they play out the heroic roles that they would be too fearful to re-create in real life, like James Thurber's character Walter Mitty. *China* is an important homeopathic medicine for weakness after blood loss and also for excitement after hearing (or imagining) horrible things, which was the central feature in Jeffrey's case.

We conferred with Jeffrey's mother by telephone two months later. Immediately after taking the medicine Jeffrey became quite hyper for four days. Then, "like magic," he exhibited greater awareness of his surroundings. Six days following his taking the *China,* Jeffrey spontaneously illustrated three pages of karate techniques. His interest in television diminished, and he began to read avidly. When his teacher asked him to read one book, he read ten. The talk about monsters stopped, and, upon his sister's request to read to him, he now selected Dr. Seuss. Jeffrey's father was amazed at his transformation. His progress continued, and within nine months he was moved to a gifted program in a mainstream classroom where he was considered one of the best students. He was selected as the most promising student in his entire school. For the first time in his life, Jeffrey now had several friends. Jeffrey's mother now mentioned that a prominent psychologist in her area had previously evaluated Jeffrey as having the profile of a serial killer.

One year after beginning homeopathic treatment, Jeffrey's conversational abilities were vastly improved. He mentioned monsters now and then, but he was more occupied with baseball and basketball. In fact, he planned to grow up to be a great basketball star or an actor. Jeffrey did so well in school that the other children asked him regularly for help with their assignments. He has needed five doses of the *China* over the past twenty-seven months, one for a setback when he moved to a new school and felt rejected by the other children. This child has blossomed even beyond his parents' hopes.

PART FOUR

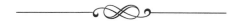

Now That You Know About Homeopathy

19

Can Homeopathy
Help *My* Child?
How to Evaluate
Whether Homeopathy
Is for Your Family

Theoretically, homeopathy should be able to help anyone. Unfortunately, as much as we would like it to be true, homeopathy does not help every child. Acknowledging this, how can you be reasonably sure that homeopathy is worth pursuing for *your* child?

Several factors are important in ensuring homeopathic success. On the homeopath's part, skill and knowledge, a well-taken case history, finding the correct medicine, and careful and accurate management of the case are essential for success. On the family's part, careful observation and reports of the child's symptoms and state, commitment to the process by both parents and child for one to two years, faith in the practitioner, patience, avoidance of interfering influences, and willingness to continue follow-up care at prescribed intervals are all necessary. Although it may seem that it is all up to the homeopath to find the medicine and cure the child, the family plays an essential role.

The Homeopath's Skill and Knowledge

Not all homeopaths are created equal. They vary in training, medical background, style of practice, and experience. Some have considerable experience treating children; others treat primarily adults. The same is true with psychiatric experience, which is highly variable. Nevertheless, the basic process of the homeopathic interview is the same for most practitioners. The mind and emotions are an essential part of every homeopathic case, and any well-trained homeopath should be able to recognize the mental patterns of most homeopathic medicines without being a psychiatrist. However, the more difficult and complicated the case, the more likely you might want to seek out a practitioner with both extensive homeopathic and psychiatric training and experience.

Because of the sheer lack of qualified homeopaths in the United States, you may not find someone who is experienced in treating behavior disorders in children in your area. You may have to travel to another state or do a telephone consultation. It is better to have an experienced practitioner work with your child, even if travel or extra expense is involved initially.

A Well-Taken Case

The beginning of the homeopathic process is the initial interview. The homeopath tries to find out everything about your child in sixty to ninety minutes. You and your child's input is essential. The better able you are to talk knowledgeably about your child's feelings, behavior, problems, interests, idiosyncrasies, and likes and dislikes, the easier it will be for her to find the correct medicine. Think about your child before the interview.

Ask your child some questions about himself. Read reports about your child from the school and psychologists. If you read the cases in this book and *Ritalin-Free Kids,* you will get some idea of the kind of information a homeopath is seeking.

Finding the Correct Medicine

Homeopathic success hinges on finding the best medicine for your child. As you can see from some of the cases in this book, a number of homeopathic medicines may be a close enough match to have some effect, but only one medicine is likely to produce a dramatic and lasting effect. Sometimes this medicine is immediately apparent. In other cases, it may take some time and research, but usually the correct medicine will be found.

Patience Is a Virtue for Homeopathic Patients

Commitment to the process is very important. Read all you can about homeopathy and what to expect from treatment. We recommend *The Patient's Guide to Homeopathic Medicine* and other books listed in the appendix for information and inspiration. An experienced homeopath is often able to select the correct medicine after the first interview, but this process can sometimes take months or, rarely, a year or more. Be patient, and expect a minimum of one to two years of treatment. If your practitioner is not having success after nine months to a year, you may wish to discuss with her the possibility of either switching to another homeopath or getting a consult from a practitioner with more experience.

The Value of Careful Follow-up

Half the challenge in homeopathic treatment is finding the correct medicine. The other half is managing the ups and downs of treatment. The family is responsible for coming for scheduled visits and supplying accurate information about progress or the lack of it.

The list of potentially antidoting substances and procedures needs to be taken seriously. It is helpful if anyone who works closely with your child, including caregivers, ex-spouses, stepparents, teachers, and housecleaners, are familiar with what needs to be avoided. If the child's symptoms return suddenly, it is likely that an interfering substance was the culprit. After the medicine is repeated and the child is doing well again, try to avoid a similar occurrence. Once the correct medicine is known, antidoting is usually an annoying setback, not a disaster, and the child generally will respond well once the medicine is repeated.

If your child relapses, please tell your homeopath. Rapid improvement will usually occur if the medicine is given soon afterward, and a lot of potential problems can be avoided. If you do not alert your homeopath to the relapse promptly, the school may be calling, your child's behavior may return to its previously rowdy and unmanageable state, and your home life may deteriorate again into chaos and discord. Your homeopath can do a much better job of managing your child's case if she has the proper information at the right time.

Come for your scheduled visits at suggested intervals. Your homeopath will intentionally allow a certain interval between office visits—enough time to thoroughly evaluate the effect of the medicine and not too much that you will have forgotten exactly what happened after your child took it. Once your child is doing better, your practitioner will begin to schedule appointments less frequently.

"Can We Really Do It? Is It Really Worth It?"

Homeopathy is natural, has much fewer side effects, and is quite a bit cheaper in the long run. However, there are some things to avoid, and you have to follow up regularly with your homeopath until your child is stably better. You and your child are likely to succeed with homeopathy if you are willing to follow the program, invest your time, energy, and money, and do what is required.

If it seems like the homeopathic process is too much for you, it may be. It takes teamwork with your homeopath and persistence to make it work. You have to evaluate the cost of treatment in terms of money, time, and effort. Conventional medicine may seem easier, even though it, too, can be quite costly and may cause potentially serious side effects.

Is it worth it? Only you can answer that question. The cases in our book are typical cases from our practice. Perhaps they remind you of your own child. The changes in those children are real. Those changes are possible for your child, too. As we mentioned previously, we estimate that 70 percent of children with behavioral problems can be helped with homeopathy if treatment is continued for at least one year. Now that you know what homeopathy has to offer, you can make an educated choice about whether this type of healing is appropriate for you and your family.

20

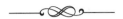

What Everyone Wants to Know About Homeopathy
Answers to the
Most Common Questions

➤ *Can homeopathy help my child with his oppositional attitude, rage, aggression, violence, or other emotional and behavioral problems?*

In many cases, homeopathy can help substantially improve or eliminate these kind of problems. However, each child is individual, so treatment results do vary. The cases in this book and our other book, *Ritalin-Free Kids* are a guide to the kinds of children homeopathy can help. If you have specific questions or reservations about whether homeopathy can help your particular child, call the homeopath's office for more information before beginning treatment.

➤ *Can I treat my own child based on the cases in your book?*

Definitely not. *Rage-Free Kids* is *not* a manual for self-treatment. We do *not* recommend self-treatment with homeopathy for *any* chronic mental, emotional, or physical condition, especially *not* serious psychiatric problems. Refer to our book, *Homeopathic Self-Care: The Quick and Easy Guide for the Whole Family* to find out about all the health problems that can be self-treated safely at home. But a competent, experienced home-opath to treat your child for the kinds of problems described in this book. If you have an insight about your child from the book, share it with your practitioner. It may open a line of inquiry that will help the homeopath find the correct medicine.

➤ *If my child's misbehavior comes from a biochemical imbalance, can homeopathy still help?*

According to homeopathic philosophy, the imbalance in biochemistry is not the *cause* of the misbehavior but rather the *result* of a fundamental imbalance in the whole person. It is the state of the child that leads to opposition, rage, aggression, and other problems. Measuring biochemical imbalances is just one way that the state can be partially known. The goal of homeopathy is to bring deep and long-lasting balance into the person's life and health rather than just to regulate serotonin, dopamine, or some other neurotransmitter or chemical. When the homeopathic medicine reduces or eliminates the child's entire set of mental, emotional, and physical symptoms or imbalances, the body's chemistry should automatically normalize as part of the overall healing process. There are rare exceptions, such as in the case of genetic deficiencies, where a specific factor must be supplemented.

➤ *How will I know whether the homeopathic medicine is working?*

Within four to eight weeks, your child will begin to feel better in general, start being less negative and angry, become more compliant and even helpful at times, and, if you are lucky, become a wonderful helper around the house. He will have fewer emotional outbursts, arguments, fights or incidences of aggression. His energy, vitality, and physical health is likely to improve as well. Your child may also have a more rapid growth or developmental spurt than is typical for him. Homeopaths generally expect at least a 70 percent improvement in many or all of the child's symptoms over time, once the correct medicine is given.

➤ *What if the first homeopathic medicine does not work?*

Your homeopath will interview you and the child again, restudy her case, and prescribe a different medicine. Don't give up on homeopathy, even if several medicines do not work. The more your homeopath learns about your child and comes to understand what works and what doesn't, the more likely he is to be able to find the correct medicine. Homeopaths do not give up easily because they know what a profound transformation the correct medicine can bring to your child's life.

➤ *If I don't think the medicine is working, why do I have to wait two months to find out?*

It takes time for the homeopathic medicine to bring about changes in your child. It took quite a while for him to get that way, and it takes less time, but still some time, for him to get better. A few children get better right away, but many have a brief period of aggravation followed by gradual, steady improvement. If you judge the medicine during the aggravation period or before the improvement gets rolling, you may be tempted to abandon it before it has time to bring about the improvement. Leaving the correct remedy prematurely will waste time for everyone. It is better to give each medicine a fair trial before moving on.

➤ *How long will my child need homeopathic treatment?*

It is best to give homeopathic treatment at least one to two years to maximize treatment gains. Although significant progress often occurs in the first one to three months, as you have seen in our cases, progress will continue to develop and stabilize over time. Many people who have discovered the substantial benefits of homeopathy choose to make it the primary source of health care for themselves and their family, consulting conventional practioners for emergencies or illnesses requiring surgery of hospitalization.

➤ *How often will my child need to see the homeopath?*

Initially, visits are scheduled every five to eight weeks. When the correct medicine has been found and the child's progress is definite and stable, visits may be only a few times a year or as needed to address new problems or maintain treatment progress.

➤ *How often will the homeopathic medicine be given?*

The simple answer is: only when necessary. Homeopathic medicines may be given in single doses, in which case the medicine will only be repeated when the original symptoms begin to return, or changed when new symptoms arise. As long as your child is responding well to the medicine she has been given, her homeopath lets the healing process proceed without redosing.

The medicines may also be prescribed to be taken on a daily or weekly basis. If your child has been given a schedule for taking the medicine, continue it as directed until your child's homeopath tells them to stop. If they run out, call the office for a refill. If you are not sure whether to keep using the medicine, call or see your practitioner.

➤ *Are there side effects from homeopathic medicines?*

Although homeopathic medicines are safe and gentle, they are capable of producing powerful changes in people. There is no equivalent reference for the side effects of homeopathic medicines such as the *Physician's Desk Reference* (PDR) for pharmaceutical drugs, primarily because the effects of homeopathic medicines are individual to the person who is taking them. A person may experience certain symptoms as part of her healing process. Both an aggravation (brief flare-up of already existing symptoms occurring within the first week of taking a homeopathic medicine) and a return of old symptoms (brief reexperiencing of symptoms that you have had in the past) can occur. Both are usually an indication that the medicine is correct for you and will usually be followed by significant improvement. Rarely, an individual may experience a new symptom after taking a homeopathic medicine. If the new symptom is troubling or severe, call your homeopath.

➤ *Can my child begin homeopathic treatment while he is still taking conventional medication?*

The answer is generally yes. Most of the time, homeopathy and conventional medicine can work together. As your child's mental, emotional, and physical health improves, it is highly likely that his prescription medications can be decreased or discontinued. This depends, of course, on many factors including the diagnosis, severity of the symptoms, and your child's unique situation. Be sure to tell your homeopath about any conventional medications your child is taking and discuss their impact on your child's homeopathic treatment and what to do about them. Some medications should not be stopped suddenly. If you wish to discontinue any medications, consult with the prescribing physician first for guidelines.

> ► *How expensive is homeopathic treatment?*

Homeopathic treatment may seem somewhat costly at first, because the homeopath has to initially spend quite a bit of time to interview and examine your child, then more time to study the case if it is complicated. The first office visit lasts from one to one and a half hours, and follow-up visits are approximately thirty minutes long. Cost depends on the location, experience, and licensure of the practitioner but usually ranges between two hundred and four hundred dollars for the first visit and seventy-five to one hundred dollars for follow-ups. The cost of the homeopathic medicine itself is negligible. A year's worth of homeopathic medicine usually costs less than one prescription of many conventional medicines.

> ► *Are there insurance companies that cover homeopathic medicine?*

The number of insurers is small but growing, as the public increasingly demands homeopathic care and insurance companies learn that homeopathic patients generally remain healthier and are much less costly to the insurance company in the long run. If your insurance provider does not yet cover homeopathic medicine, let the company know you want coverage for homeopathic care or find another provider. Many homeopaths do not choose to work within the insurance system for a variety of reasons. These include a desire to ensure the privacy of the patient, inadequate reimbursement for extended office visits, and a desire to operate one's practice independently rather than under the confines of a managed care system.

> *Many of the children in your cases sound worse than my child, thank God. Can homeopathy work for kids who aren't so extreme?*

Homeopathy can benefit all kinds of children, extreme or not, and their parents, too. Those children whose symptoms are very intense tend to need medicines made from more intense animal substances in nature, such as rattlesnake, scorpion, rabies, and tarantula, or psychoactive plants, such as deadly nightshade, henbane, and datura. Other milder, more even-tempered people may need gentler medicines such as those made from flowers or mineral salts.

> *Can homeopathic medicines made from toxic substances ever poison the people taking them?*

Never. Arsenic, snake venom, strychnine, and rabies are all homeopathic medicines, but they are absolutely nontoxic. The medicines carry the pattern of the original substance but, if tested, would never contain enough of the substance to be toxic or dangerous. Homeopathic medicines are diluted so many times that the original substance is absent from all but the lowest potencies. Even a 6C potency, which is quite low, only carries one part per hundred million of the original substance.

> *What is the difference between taking a single homeopathic medicine and the combination homeopathic medicines that I have seen in my health food store?*

Only one homeopathic medicine at any point in time will have a complete and dramatic effect on your healing. An experienced homeopathic practitioner is trained to find that one specific medicine that most closely matches your symptoms and that can produce profound, lasting healing. Combination medicines contain a variety of common homeopathic substances that have been found useful for a certain condition such as a cold, flu, or sore throat. If the one medicine that you need is contained in that combination, you will be healed. If not, you will have little or no response to the medicine. We recommend taking one medicine at a time for the best results.

Combination medicines should only be used for acute conditions when you cannot identify the one medicine that best matches the symptom picture or when no qualified homeopath is available. They should not be used for chronic or recurring conditions such as ADHD, conduct disorder, oppositional defiant disorder, and the other conditions mentioned in this book. The same is true of chronic physical ailments such as asthma, headaches, eczema, and arthritis. For chronic disease, find a trained homeopath, and you will be much more likely to be helped safely, effectively, and often dramatically by homeopathy.

➤ *How long do I need to avoid the substances and influences that interfere with homeopathic treatment?*

Follow your homeopath's instructions regarding what to avoid. It is important to avoid these items as long as you are being treated homeopathically. Symptoms have returned after exposure to such influences for as much as two years after taking the homeopathic medicine. If you have been helped significantly by homeopathy, it is probably best to play it safe and continue to avoid such exposure indefinitely. Individual sensitivity varies, however, and some items on the list may not be a problem for you. The difficulty is knowing which will cause a relapse and which will not. If your child suddenly relapses, even years after treatment, call or see your homeopath for reevaluation. Consistent follow-up with your homeopath will help avoid any unnecessary ups and downs in treatment.

➤ *What if I or my child has food or environmental allergies?*

Homeopathy treats the whole child, including her allergies. When your child is given a homeopathic medicine that closely matches her symptoms and state, her immune system will become stronger and less susceptible to allergens. It is typical for patients who respond well to homeopathy to be able eventually to go back to eating or being exposed to substances that bothered them prior to homeopathic treatment, without their former allergic responses. At times a homeopathic medicine can be prescribed to alleviate acute allergic reactions such as hives or hay fever.

➤ *I can't get my son to stop eating junk food. Will homeopathy still work for him?*

Even though most children are better in general from a healthy diet, and it is much healthier for children to eat fresh, whole foods and to avoid the empty calories found in high-sugar, high-fat, and processed foods, the right homeopathic medicine will still be effective for junk-food addicts.

➤ *How can I find a qualified homeopath in my area?*

See "Referral Sources for Homeopathic Practitioners" in the appendix.

➤ *How do I know whether my local homeopath practices the same way you describe in your book?*

Ask the homeopath whether she practices classical homeopathy. A classical homeopath uses one medicine at a time and spends at least one hour with the patient during the initial interview. Ask where the practitioner was trained. It should be an extensive course with a bare minimum of five hundred hours and, preferably, two years or more, in addition to ongoing seminars, conferences, and training. Find out how long the person has been practicing homeopathy and what percentage of his or her practice is homeopathy. The longer in practice, and the more time devoted to homeopathy, the better. Look for a homeopath who graduated from an accredited or well-respected program of training and who devotes a minimum of 50 percent of her practice to homeopathy. If you are looking for the type of treatment that we discuss in this book, we do not recommend practitioners who select medicines by using machines, pendulums, or muscle testing.

➤ *What if there is no experienced homeopath in my area?*
We are very willing to treat patients by telephone. Some other homeopaths do also, while others insist on in-person visits, either the first time or during the entire course of treatment. Exactly the same interview process is involved. It is almost the same as visiting the homeopath in person. We interview both the parent and the child over the phone. We have personally found the results are generally just as good as conducting the interview in our office. When a physical examination is needed, we ask our patient to consult with a local physician. We function as specialists. If you are uncomfortable working with your homeopath by telephone, you can also choose a practitioner in a neighboring city or state. This is not as impractical as with conventional medical care since the visits are relatively infrequent—between every six weeks to six months.

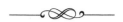

A New Millennium
The Time Has Come for
Homeopathy to Flourish

We doubt there is anyone who would question that violence and aggression among children is a serious problem worthy of tremendous attention, concern, research, and action. Also evident is that many of the existing answers, for a variety of reasons, do not offer meaningful and lasting results. One reason for treatment failure is lack of compliance. "Dropping out from treatment is a significant problem in the treatment of children and adolescents. Among families that begin treatment, 40 to 60 percent terminate prematurely. Youths with aggressive and antisocial behavior are particularly likely to drop out early."[1] However, even when parent and child are quite reliable with treatment, there is no one simple answer for helping violent and aggressive kids.

We need to address this situation on many different levels: the individual child; family; classroom; the educational, medical, mental health, and criminal justice systems; and the local and federal government. Certainly answers lie in all of these different spheres. It is the task of educators to explore how best to teach our children; of parents to best meet the needs of their growing children in a challenging world; of physicians, con ventional and alternative, to work together to discover the best therapeutic interventions for these kids; of mental health professionals to develop effective and meaningful strategies that can help turn children's lives in a positive direction; of criminal justice professionals to find alternatives to incarceration that increase rehabilitation and decrease recidivism; and of sociologists, social workers, and legislators to create systems to increase wealth and opportunities for all and to regulate programming for children and availability of weapons. There are more than enough tasks for everyone in the effort to curb childhood violence.

We need to remember that the solutions come in many different forms. Take, for example, an impressive feature article that appeared recently in the *Seattle Times*: The Reverend Reggie Witherspoon welcomes anyone, no matter how they look or what they've done, into his church. One of Witherspoon's prominent mentors, Tim McGee, was once a notorious gang member ticketed for a short life. Now McGee prays so hard he almost cries as the congregation worships exuberantly. At first the dynamic minister, who lost his own brother to a violent murder, found himself presiding over the funerals of young gang members in the neighborhood. Witherspoon ultimately earned their respect, some turned over their guns to him, and the African American boys, perhaps 70 percent of whom were fatherless, began to pack the church. Now the nine-hundred-strong church, with the help of a congregation member and account, has established a nonprofit community development corporation which attracts loan, grants, and donations to help teen mothers, the homeless, youth programs, and financial planning services. Witherspoon has found a moving way to turn kids from crime to God.[3] Right on, Reverend Reggie!

A Number of Solutions Have Been Suggested

A Brown University symposium collected recommendations from respected experts in the field of violence in adolescents and children. They made the following excellent suggestions:[2]

- Take a collective moral responsibility for violence and make a long-term, national commitment to its eradication.
- Shift from a reactive to a proactive stance.
- Treat violence as a public health issue like smoking.
- Support health care reform efforts and funding for intervention and assessment services.
- Practice prevention; reach kids as early as possible.
- Teach nonviolent conflict resolution to everyone.
- Ban handguns.
- Ban corporal punishment.
- Restrict media violence and promote responsible children's television programming.
- Invest money and programs in communities at risk for violence.
- Start a national day care program that includes parent education.
- Create more jobs and vocational programs.
- Coordinate communication among kids, parents, schools, police, and communities.
- Coordinate social and medical services within schools.

Alternative Medicine Is on the Move

There is also no question that alternative medicine is no longer a secret. In a recent interview, Wayne Jonas, M.D., departing director of the Office of Alternative Medicine, recently renamed the National Center for Complementary and Alternative Medicine, was asked, "Are you hopeful about the direction of alternative medicine in the next millennium?" Dr. Jonas replied, "I don't think you have to be hopeful. You can see it happening before your eyes right now. It's not a sideline of American medicine. It's an important main part of American medicine. I think we'll see a new integrated type of health care system as we enter the next millennium."[4]

Homeopathy is widely accepted in Europe, by physicians, patients, and the public. There is no doubt that the trend is growing here as well. Homeopathic medicine is more elegant than herbs or nutrition, but harder for many to comprehend. As more and more people are able to clearly distinguish the difference between homeopathy and other forms of alternative medicine and to see for themselves the profound changes that can occur by simply giving one medicine (the right medicine, of course) at a time, the demand for homeopathic care cannot help but rise exponentially. That is already beginning to happen.

Getting to the Roots of the Problem

Peggy O'Mara, pioneering editor of *Mothering* magazine, in a frank editorial entitled "Kids Who Kill" penetrated the heart of the problem of violence in kids.

> Recent shooting sprees and murders of schoolchildren by other children shock us. We weep for the victims and are incredulous of the assailants. We simply cannot understand the out-of-control, premeditated behavior of violent children. How does

conscience develop? . . . It is the byproduct of a healthy attachment process in infancy. If we attach securely to one consistent caregiver in the first three years of life, we develop affection. . . . It is not that guns and television shows have made us a violent society; rather it is that they are products of our violence. Anthropologists have found among indigenous peoples worldwide a correlation between violence in adulthood and lack of touch in infancy. . . . Holding and touching our infants and children is perhaps the most important thing we can do to ensure their normal neurological and psychological development. . . . We can't control the fates of our children, but we can raise them in a nonviolent way. We can learn the signs of trouble in young people with impaired consciences. We can work for the modeling of less violence in society as depicted in the media. We can debate guns seriously without special interests. And, we can be a society that helps parents, that loves children, that does everything possible to ensure healthy families.[5]

We couldn't agree more that the ultimate cause of violence is children (or adults, for that matter) feeling separate, isolated, alone, and unloved. It is only by separating oneself from one's fellow beings on the planet that it is possible to even contemplate killing, much less doing so without remorse. Without such depersonalization, tragedies like those in Jonesboro, Springfield, and Littleton would never occur.

May All Be Healed

Whether it be through homeopathy, a system that we have found to be effective for so many who are suffering, or through any other approach, we hope that the victims and perpetrators of violence, as well as all those whose lives are affected by their actions, may find healing— that, even in seemingly the darkest of hearts, love and peace may prevail.

Appendix: Learning More

Recommended Books

Violence and Other Behavioral Problems in Children

Barkley, Russell. *Attention Deficit Hyperactivity Disorder: A Handbook for Diagnosis and Treatment.* New York: Guilford, 1990.

Canfield, Jack, et al. *Chicken Soup for the Kid's Soul.* Deerfield Beach, FL: Health Communications, 1998.

———. *Chicken Soup for the Teenage Soul.* Deerfield Beach, FL: Health Communications, 1997.

———. *Chicken Soup for the Teenage Soul II.* Deerfield Beach, FL: Health Communications, 1998.

Carter, William Lee. *The Angry Teenager.* Nashville: Nelson, 1995.

Edwards, C. Drew. *How to Handle a Hard-to-Handle Kid: A Parent's Guide to Understanding and Changing Problem Behaviors.* Minneapolis: Free Spirit, 1999.

Faber, Adele, and Elain Mazlish. *How to Talk So Kids Will Listen & Listen So Kids Will Talk.* New York: Avon, 1980.

Ford, Judy. *Wonderful Ways to Be a Family.* Berkeley, CA: Conari, 1998.

———. *Wonderful Ways to Love a Child.* Berkeley, CA: Conari, 1994.

———. *Wonderful Ways to Love a Teen—Even When It Seems Impossible.* Berkeley, CA: Conari, 1996.

Forehand, Rex, and Nicholas Long. *Parenting the Strong-Willed Child.* Lincolnwood, IL: NTC, 1996.

Fruge, Ernest, and Christine Adams. *Why Children Misbehave and What to Do about It.* Oakland, CA: New Harbinger, 1996.

Golant, Mitch, and Donna Corwin. *The Challenging Child: A Guide for Parents of Exceptionally Strong-Willed Children.* New York: Berkeley, 1995.

Green, Rose. *The Explosive Child.* New York: HarperCollins, 1998.

Hartmann, Thom. *ADD Success Stories.* Grass Valley, CA: Underwood, 1995.

————. *Attention Deficit Disorder: A Different Perspective.* Novato, CA: Underwood-Miller, 1993.

Heide, Kathleen. *Why Kids Kill Parents.* Thousand Oaks, CA: Sage, 1992.

Hewlett, Sylvia, and Cornell West. *The War Against Parents: What We Can Do for America's Beleaguered Moms and Dads.* New York: Mariner Books, 1998.

Karr-Morse, Robin, and Meredith Wiley. *Ghosts in the Nursery: Tracing the Roots of Violence.* New York: Atlantic Monthly Press, 1997.

LeShan, Eda. *When Your Child Drives You Crazy.* New York: St. Martin's, 1985.

Levinson, Kathy. *First Aid for Tantrums.* Boca Raton, FL: Saturn, 1997.

Lynn, George. *Survival Strategies for Parenting Your ADD Child.* Grass Valley, CA: Underwood, 1996.

McKay, Matthew, et al. *When Anger Hurts Your Kids: A Parents' Guide.* Oakland, CA: New Harbinger, 1996.

Siegel, Bryna. *The World of the Autistic Child: Understanding and Treating Autistic Spectrum Disorder.* New York: Oxford University Press, 1996.

Smith, Romayne, editor. *Children with Mental Retardation: A Parents' Guide.* Bethesda, MD: Woodbine House, 1993.

Sullivan, Tom. *Special Parent, Special Child.* New York: Tarcher & Putnam, 1995.

Wilens, Timothy, M.D. *Straight Talk about Psychiatric Medications for Kids.* New York: Guilford, 1998.

Homeopathy

Bellavite, Paolo, and Andrea Signorini. *Homeopathy: A Frontier in Medical Science.* Berkeley: North Atlantic, 1995.

Castro, Miranda. *Homeopathic Guide to Stress.* New York: St. Martin's Griffin, 1997.

Grossinger, Richard. *Homeopathy: The Great Riddle.* Berkeley: North Atlantic Press, 1980.

Jonas, Wayne, and Jennifer Jacobs. *Healing with Homeopathy.* New York: Warner, 1996.

Reichenberg-Ullman, Judyth, and Robert Ullman. *Prozac-Free: Homeopathic Medicine for Depression, Anxiety and Other Mental and Emotional Problems.* Rocklin, CA: Prima, 1999.

Reichenberg-Ullman, Judyth, and Robert Ullman. *Ritalin-Free Kids: Safe and Effective Homeopathic Medicine for ADD and Other Behavioral and Learning Problems.* Rocklin, CA: Prima, 1996.

Ullman, Dana. *The Consumer's Guide to Homeopathic Medicine.* New York: Tarcher/Putnam, 1995.

Ullman, Robert, and Judyth Reichenberg-Ullman. *Homeopathic Self-Care: The Quick and Easy Guide for the Whole Family.* Rocklin, CA: Prima Publishing, 1997.

Ullman, Robert, and Judyth Reichenberg-Ullman. *The Patient's Guide to Homeopathic Medicine.* Edmonds, WA: Picnic Point Press, 1995.

Homeopathic Book Distributors

Homeopathic Educational
Services
2124 Kittredge St.
Berkeley, CA 94704
(510) 649-0294 (for inquiries or catalogues)
(800) 359-9051 (orders only)

The Minimum Price
250 H St., PO Box 2187
Blaine, WA 98231
(800) 663-8272

Referral Sources for Homeopathic Practitioners

Homeopathic practitioners vary widely regarding level of medical or psychiatric training and experience, licensing or certification, expertise, and style of practice. Not all of the practitioners in the following directories necessarily use the same methods we have described in this book or are qualified to treat patients with serious mental illness.

Homeopathic Academy of
Naturopathic Physicians
(HANP)
12132 SE Foster Place
Portland, OR 97266
Telephone: (503) 761-3298
Fax: (503) 762-1929

The National Center for
Homeopathy (NCH)
801 N. Fairfax, #306
Alexandria, VA 22314
Telephone: (703) 548-7790
Fax: (703) 548-7792

Council for Homeopathic
Certification (CHC)
P.O. Box 460190
San Francisco, CA 94146
(415) 789-7677

American Institute of
Homeopathy (AIH)
10418 Whithead St.
Fairfax, VA 22030
(703) 246-9501

North American Society of
Homeopaths (NASH)
1122 East Pike St.,
Suite 1122
Seattle, WA 98122
(206) 720-7000

Glossary

affective disorder—a derangement of mood as in depression, anxiety, or bipolar disorder

aggravation—a temporary worsening of already existing symptoms after taking a homeopathic medicine

allopathic medicine—a type of medicine, unlike homeopathy, which uses a different, rather than a similar, medicine to heal a set of symptoms

alternative medicine—natural approaches to healing that are nontoxic and safe, including homeopathy, naturopathic medicine, chiropractic, acupuncture, botanical medicine, and many other methods of healing

antidepressant—a substance that alleviates depression

antidote—a substance or influence that interferes with homeopathic treatment

antipsychotic—a prescription medication used to treat patients with schizophrenia and other thought disorders

antisocial personality disorder—a recurrent pattern of disregard for and violation of the rights of others

Asperger's disorder—a type of pervasive developmental disorder, sometimes called a high-functioning form of autism, characterized by impaired eye contact, failure to develop appropriate peer relationships, and a lack of ability to establish social or emotional contact

attention deficit/hyperactivity disorder (ADHD or ADD)—a diagnosis based on a constellation of symptoms that includes attention problems, impulsivity, and/or hyperactivity

autism or autistic disorder—a type of pervasive developmental disorder characterized by delayed social interaction, language or play; repetitive and stereotyped behavior; and difficulty in communication and social interaction

bipolar disorder—a mood disorder, formerly known as manic depression, characterized by episodes of fluctuating moods ranging from depression to mania

borderline personality disorder—a pattern of instability of interpersonal relations, impulsivity, disturbed identity, and recurrent suicidal gestures or threats

case taking—the process of the in-depth homeopathic interview

chief complaint—the main problem that causes a patient to visit a health care practitioner

classical homeopathy—a method of homeopathic prescribing in which only one medicine is given at a time based on the totality of the patient's symptoms elicited in an in-depth interview

combination medicine—a mixture containing more than one homeopathic medicine

conduct disorder (CD)—a repetitive and persistent behavioral pattern in which the basic rights of others and of societal norms or rules are violated

constitutional treatment—homeopathic treatment based on the whole person, involving an extensive interview and careful follow-up

conventional medicine—mainstream, orthodox, Western medicine

defense mechanism—the aspect of the vital force that maintains health and prevents disease

depression—a mood disorder characterized by persistent feelings of hopelessness accompanied by appetite changes, sleep problems, low energy or fatigue, and impaired self-esteem

developmental disability—mental or physical delays in development or maturity due to genetic or congenital abnormalities; also called mental retardation

disruptive behavior disorder—a group of diagnoses manifested by behavioral patterns that are disruptive to others, including attention deficit/hyperactivity disorder, oppositional defiant disorder, and conduct disorder

dissociative identity disorder (formerly multiple personality disorder)—the presence of two or more identities or personality states, each with its own pattern of perceiving and thinking

DSM-IV—officially recognized diagnostic manual of mental and emotional conditions published by the American Psychiatric Association

FDA—U.S. Food and Drug Administration

high-potency medicines—homeopathic medicines of a 200C or higher potency

homeopathic medicine—a medicine that acts according to the principles of homeopathy

homeopathic practitioner—a practitioner who treats people with homeopathic medicines according to the principles of homeopathic medicine as developed by Samuel Hahnemann

homeopathy—a medical science and art that treats the whole person based on the principle of like cures like

law of similars—the principle of like cures like

low-potency medicines—homeopathic medicines of a 30C or lower potency

materia medica—a book that includes individual homeopathic medications and their indications

mental retardation—mental or physical delays in development or maturity due to genetic or congenital abnormalities; also called developmental disability

minimum dose—the least quantity of a medicine that produces a change in a person who is ill

modality—those factors that make a particular symptom better or worse

mother tincture—an extract of the original substance from which a homeopathic medicine is made

naturopathic physician—a physician who has graduated from a four-year naturopathic medical school and who treats the whole person based on the principle of the healing power of nature

neurotransmitter—a chemical substance, such as serotonin or dopamine, that transmits nerve impulses in the brain and nervous system, affecting thinking, behavior, and sensory and motor function

nosode—a homeopathic medicine made from the products of disease

obsessive compulsive disorder—a diagnostic category that includes symptoms of obsessive thought patterns and ritualistic behaviors

oppositional-defiant disorder (ODD)—a pattern of negative and defiant behavior involving argumentativeness, resentment, vindictiveness, and abdication of personal responsibility

panic attack—an episode of extreme anxiety typified by a racing heart, perspiration, hyperventilation, lightheadedness, apprehension, and fear

pervasive developmental disorder—impairment in social interaction characterized by limited eye contact, difficulty developing relationships with peers, delayed or limited communication, and stereotyped or repetitive behaviors

phobia—an unreasonable, out of proportion, persistent fear of a specific thing

posttraumatic stress disorder—the persistent reexperiencing of a past traumatic event in the form of recollections, dreams, or flashbacks

potency—the strength of a homeopathic medicine as determined by the number of serial dilutions and succussions

potentization—the preparation of a homeopathic medicine through the process of serial dilution and succussion

prover—a person who takes a specific homeopathic substance as part of a specially designed homeopathic experiment to test the action of the medicine

provings—the process of testing out homeopathic substances in a prescribed way to understand their potential curative action on patients

relapse—the return of symptoms when a homeopathic medicine is no longer acting

repertory—a book that lists symptoms and the medicines known to produce such symptoms in healthy provers or in clinical practice

return of old symptoms—the reexperiencing of symptoms from the past, after taking a homeopathic medicine, as part of the healing process

schizophrenia—a thought disorder characterized by confusion, disorientation, delusions, and hallucinations

serotonin—a neurotransmitter in the brain that can affect moods and behavior

simillimum—the one homeopathic medicine that most clearly matches the symptoms of the patient and that produces the greatest benefit

single medicine—one single homeopathic medicine given at a time

SSRI— selective serotonin reuptake inhibitor; one of a family of antidepressants that increase levels of serotonin in the brain

state—an individual's stance in life; how she or he approaches the world

succussion—the systematic and repeated shaking of a homeopathic medicine after each serial dilution

symptom picture—a constellation of all of the mental, emotional, and physical symptoms that an individual patient experiences

thought disorder—derangement of cognitive processes, as in schizophrenia

tic disorder—a symptom picture characterized by twitches, jerks, and other convulsive or uncontrollable behaviors

totality—a comprehensive picture of the whole person: physical, mental, and emotional

traumatic brain injury—a head injury resulting in neurological damage to the brain

vital force—the invisible energy present in all living things that creates harmony, balance, and health

Notes

Introduction

1. "Boy Attacks Mother over Nintendo Game," *Seattle Times*, February 26, 1998, B2.
2. Kyle Wood, "Many Dangers Face Kids Raised Here, Study Says," *Seattle Times,* September 23, 1996, B1.
3. Peggy O'Mara, "An Epidemic of Violence." *Mothering* 95 (July/August 1999): 6.
4. Daniel Connor and Ronald Steingard, "A Clinical Approach to the Pharmacotherapy of Aggression in Children and Adolescents," *Annals New York Academy of Sciences* 794 (September 20, 1996): 290.
5. Kathleen Heide, *Why Kids Kill Parents: Child Abuse and Adolescent Homicide* (Thousand Oaks, CA: Sage, 1992), 3.
6. Samuel Maull, "Jury Convicts Man in Death of New York City Teacher," *Seattle Times,* November 11, 1998, A4.
7. Gary Zinik, "Letters: Jury Still Out on Whether Killers Are Born or Made. Nature vs. Nurture: U.S. School Shootings Have Left 14 People Dead and 26 Injured Since Oct. 1," *Ventura County Star* (Ventura, CA) July 29, 1998, B7.
8. Myriam Miedzian, "Unlinking the Chain of Teen Violence," *Chicago Tribune,* June 12, 1998, 23.
9. Geoffry Cowley and Anne Underwood, "What's Alternative?" *Newsweek,* November 23, 1998, 68.
10. Brenda Paik Sunoo, "On a Solid Foundation: A Conversation with Wayne B. Jonas, the Departing Director of

NCCAM," *Alternative Healthcare Management* (January 1999): 24.

Chapter 1

1. David Stout, "Clinton Is 'Profoundly Shocked' by Tragedy," *Seattle Post-Intelligencer,* April 21, 1999, A12.
2. Mike Anton, "Up to 25 Killed in Rampage," *Seattle Post-Intelligencer,* April 21, 1999, A1; and Robin McDowell, "'Trench Coat Mafia' a Dark Presence at School," *Seattle Post-Intelligencer,* April 21, 1999, A12.
3. Jerry M. Weiner, editor, *Textbook of Child and Adolescent Psychiatry* (Washington, D.C.: American Psychiatric Press, 1991), 277–278.
4. Dana Oland, "Violence: Shooting in Oregon Brings Problem Closer to Home," *Idaho Statesman,* June 2,1998, 1d.
5. Ray Suarez, "Jonesboro Convictions," National Public Radio, *Talk of the Nation,* August 12, 1998.
6. Dawn Chmielewski and Leslie Gornstein, "The Issue of Violent Video Games Is a New Quandary for Parents," *Houston Chronicle,* 2 Star Edition, December 3, 1998, 2.
7. Ibid.
8. Kyle Wood, "Many Dangers Face Kids Raised Here, Study Says," *Seattle Times,* September 23, 1996, B1.
9. Lyndon Hogg, "BB Gun Shot Leads to Suspension," *Daily Post* (Rotorua, New Zealand), February 25, 1999, 3.
10. Ian Murray, "Criminal Tendencies Evident in Childhood," *The Times* (London), January 16, 1998, Home News Section, editorial.
11. Stephen Scott, "Aggressive Behaviour in Childhood," *British Medical Journal* 316 (January 17, 1998): 203.
12. Ibid., 202.
13. Madhu Jain and Ramesh Vinayak, "Children: Growing Up in Anger," *India Today* (July 27, 1998): 66.
14. Tad Dickens, "Vandalism Mars Area Schools: Incidents Occur at Any Time during the Year and the Costs Are

Adding Up," *Virginian-Pilot* (Norfolk, VA), November 11, 1998, B3.

15. Ronald Fitten, "Psychologist: Boy Meant No Harm as He Set Man Afire—Mental Illness Does Not Excuse Act, Expert Testifies," *Seattle Times,* September 18, 1997, B3.

16. "14-Year-Old Boy Is Charged in Slaying of 8-Year-Old Girl," *Seattle Times,* November 11, 1998, A4.

17. Terence Monmaney and Greg Krikorian, "Violent Culture, Media Share Blame, Experts Say; Killings: Spate of Deaths Prompts Many Explanations Including Emergence of 'Fledgling Psychopaths,'" *Los Angeles Times,* March 26, 1998, A16.

18. J. Adler and Peter Annin, "Murder at an Early Age," *Newsweek,* August 14, 1998, 28.

Chapter 2

1. Tamra Fitzpatrick, "'Bad' Kids Helped to Get Better," *Seattle Times,* December 27, 1998, B1.

2. Jerry M. Weiner, editor, *Textbook of Child and Adolescent Psychiatry* (Washington, D.C.: American Psychiatric Press, 1991), 302.

3. David Comings, "Genetic Aspects of Childhood Behavioral Disorders," *Child Psychiatry and Human Development* 27, no. 3 (Spring 1997): 148.

4. Ibid., 142.

5. Douglas Langbehn, Remi Cadoret, William Yates, Edward Troughton, and Mark Stewart, "Distinct Contributions of Conduct and Oppositional Defiant Symptoms to Adult Antisocial Behavior: Evidence from an Adoption Study," *Archives of General Psychiatry* 55 (September 1998): 821.

6. Weiner, *Textbook,* 284.

7. Dee J. Hall, "'Bad' Child May Be Mentally Ill; Society Is Just Waking Up to Scope of the Problem," *Wisconsin State Journal,* July 5, 1998, 1A.

8. Daniel Connor and Ronald Steingard, "A Clinical Approach to the Pharmacotherapy of Aggression in Children and Adolescents," *Annals New York Academy of Sciences* 794 (September 20, 1996): 291–301.

9. Carina Evens and Ann Vander Stoep, "Risk Factors for Juvenile Justice System Referral among Children in a Public Mental Health System," *Juvenile Justice Referral II, The Journal of Mental Health Administration* 24, no. 4 (Fall 1997): 451.

10. Ibid., 453.

11. Weiner, *Textbook,* 300.

12. Leslie Sowers, "The Mental Health of Children Part III. Too Late for Help? Is Incarceration the Answer?" *Houston Chronicle,* August 9, 1998, 7.

13. Maurizio Fava, "Psychopharmacologic Treatment of Pathologic Aggression," *Psychiatric Clinics of North America* 20, no. 2 (June 1997): 428.

14. Weiner, *Textbook,* 290.

15. Ibid., 291.

16. Ibid., 292.

17. Evens and Vander Stoep, "Risk Factors," 449.

18. Weiner, *Textbook,* 284.

19. Kathleen Heide, *Why Kids Kill Parents: Child Abuse and Adolescent Homicide* (Thousand Oaks, CA: Sage, 1992), 3.

20. Ibid., 6.

21. David Hall and Margaret Lynch, "Violence Begins at Home," *British Medical Journal* 316 (May 23, 1998): 1551.

22. Madhu Jain and Ramesh Vinayak, "Children: Growing Up in Anger," *India Today* (July 27, 1998): 66.

23. Judyth Reichenberg-Ullman and Robert Ullman, *Prozac-Free: Homeopathic Medicine for Depression, Anxiety and Other Mental and Emotional Problems* (Rocklin, CA: Prima, 1999), 245.

24. David Schwartz, Kenneth Dodge, Gregory Pettit, and John Bates, "The Early Socialization of Aggressive Victims of

Bullying," *Child Development* 68, no. 4 (August 1997): 665.

25. Weiner, *Textbook,* 324.
26. David Finkelhor and Lucy Berliner, "Research on the Treatment of Sexually Abused Children: A Review and Recommendations," *Journal of the American Academy of Child and Adolescent Psychiatry* 34, no. 11 (November 1995): 1408.
27. K. C. Burke et al., "Age at Onset of Selected Mental Disorders in Five Community Populations," *Archives of General Psychiatry* 47: 511–518.
28. Duncan Clark et al., "Gender and Comorbid Psychopathology in Adolescents With Alcohol Dependence," *Journal of the American Academy of Child and Adolescent Psychiatry* 36, no. 9 (September 1997): 1195.
29. Howard Moss and Levent Kirisci, "Aggressivity in Adolescent Alcohol Abusers: Relationship with Conduct Disorder," *Alcoholism Clinical and Experimental Research* 19, no. 3 (June 1995): 645.
30. Clark et al., "Gender," 1195–1196.
31. C. Ray Hall, "Our Schools' Lost Innocence: Is Violent Pop Culture Holding Kids Hostage?" *Courier-Journal* (Louisville, KY), December 6, 1998, 01X.
32. Lewis P. Lipsitt, editor, *Violence: Its Causes and Cures; The Brown University Child and Adolescent Behavior Letter* (Providence, RI: Manisses Communications Group, 1994), 11.
33. Earnestine Willis and Victor Strasburger, "Media Violence," *Pediatric Clinics of North America* 45, no. 2 (April 1998): 319.
34. Ibid., 328.
35. Terence Monmaney and Greg Krikorian, "Violent Culture, Media Share Blame, Experts Say; Killings: Spate of Deaths Prompts Many Explanations Including Emergency of 'Fledgling Psychopaths,'" *Los Angeles Times,* March 26, 1998, A16.

36. Willis and Strasberger, "Media Violence," 319–321.
37. Ibid., 324.
38. Jain and Vinayak, "Children," 66.
39. Dawn Chmielewski and Leslie Gornstein, "The Issue of Violent Video Games Is a New Quandary for Parents," *Houston Chronicle,* 2 Star Edition (December 3,1998): 2.
40. Willis and Strasberger, "Media Violence, 325.
41. Peggy O'Mara, "An Epidemic of Violence," *Mothering* 95 (July/August 1999): 8.
42. Wendy McKellips, "Students Look Elsewhere During TV Turnoff Week," *South Whidbey Record,* April 21, 1999, A9.
43. Lipsett, *Violence,* 2.
44. Ibid.
45. "Parents of Slain Students Sue Entertainment Firms," *Seattle Times,* April 13, 1999, A4.
46. Lipsett, *Violence,* 32.
47. Willis and Strasburger, "Media Violence," 327.
48. Ibid., 34.
49. O'Mara, "An Epidemic," 7.
50. Ibid., 7.
51. Lipsett, *Violence,* 16.

Chapter 3

1. Hoda Kotbe, "Breaking Point? Hidden Cameras Show One Child's Extreme Misbehavior and What His Parents Did to Correct the Problem," *Dateline NBC,* October 25, 1998.
2. Suzy Frisch, "Parents of Caged Girl Sentenced to 1 Year," *Chicago Tribune,* September 12, 1998, 8.

Chapter 4

1. Charles Schwarzbeck, "Look Beneath Surface of Behavior When Treating Troubled Children," *Houston Chronicle,* June 2, 1998, 2.

Chapter 5

1. Dee J. Hall, "'Bad' Child May Be Mentally Ill; Society Is Just Waking Up to Scope of the Problem," *Wisconsin State Journal,* July 5, 1998, 1A.
2. Daniel Connor and Ronald Steingard, "A Clinical Approach to the Pharmacotherapy of Aggression in Children and Adolescents," *Annals New York Academy of Sciences* 794 (September 20, 1996): 290.
3. Ibid., 291.
4. Ibid.
5. Timothy Wilens, M.D., *Straight Talk about Psychiatric Medications for Kids* (New York: Guilford, 1998).
6. Ibid., 174–175.
7. Connor and Steingard, "A Clinical Approach," 296.
8. Ibid., 298.
9. Wilens, *Straight Talk,* 154.
10. Connor and Steingard, "A Clinical Approach," 295.
11. Ibid., 299.
12. Kyle Wood, "Many Dangers Face Kids Raised Here, Study Says," *Seattle Times,* September 23, 1996, B1.
13. Connor and Steingard, "A Clinical Approach," 302.
14. Wilens, *Straight Talk,* 209.
15. Ibid., 212.
16. Ibid., 215.
17. Ibid., 232.

Chapter 6

1. Paul Kleinjnen, Paul Knipshild, and Gerber ter Riet, "Clinical Trials of Homeopathy." *British Medical Journal* 302 (9 February 1991): 316.

Chapter 10

1. Leslie Sowers, "Too Late to Help?: The Mental Health of Children, Teaching Discipline; Positive Learning Climate

Limits Need for Punishment," *Houston Chronicle,* May 17, 1998, 6.

Chapter 11

1. Tamra Fitzpatrick, "'Bad' Kids Helped to Get Better," *Seattle Times,* December 27, 1998, B1.
2. Ibid., B1–B2.
3. "'Rudolph' Lyrics Are Definitely Eye Opener for Boy's Parents," *Seattle Times,* December 9,1998, A3.
4. Jeff Nichols, "Second Chances: Horizon House Gives Troubled Children Last Hope for Success," *Post and Courier* (Charleston, SC), October 5, 1997, E1.
5. "To Reduce Discipline Problems, Train Teachers to Deal with Student Anger," *School Violence Alert,* Teacher Training Section 3, no. 6 (June 1997).
6. Leslie Sowers, "The Mental Health of Children Part III. Too Late for Help? Is Incarceration the Answer?" *Houston Chronicle,* August 9, 1998, 1.
7. "Washington," *USA Today,* April 24, 1998, 15A.
8. Sowers, "The Mental Health," 1.

Chapter 12

1. Geoffry Cowley and Anne Underwood, "What's Alternative?" *Newsweek,* November 23, 1998, 68.
2. Ibid.
3. Judyth Reichenberg-Ullman and Robert Ullman, *Ritalin-Free Kids: Safe and Effective Homeopathic Medicine for ADD and Other Behavioral and Learning Problems* (Rocklin, CA: Prima Publishing, 1996), 65.
4. Ibid., 65–66; Judyth Reichenberg-Ullman and Robert Ullman. *Prozac-Free: Homeopathic Medicine for Depression, Anxiety and Other Mental and Emotional Problems* (Rocklin, CA: Prima Publishing, 1999), 245.

5. Klaus Linde et al., "Are the Clinical Effects of Home-opathy Placebo Effects? A Meta-Analysis of Placebo-Controlled Trials," *Lancet* 350 (1997): 834–843.

Chapter 13

1. Rolf Loeber and Dale Hay, "Key Issues in the Develop-ment of Aggression and Violence from Childhood to Early Adulthood," *Annual Review of Psychology* 48 (1997): 374.
2. Ibid.

Chapter 14

1. Leslie Sowers, "Up to the Schools; The Mental Health of Children: Part II. Rx for Help? Medicine Becoming Com-mon Treatment for Kids' Problems," *Houston Chronicle,* June 28, 1998, 6.
2. Daniel Connor and Ronald Steingard, "A Clinical Ap-proach to the Pharmacotherapy of Aggression in Children and Adolescents," *Annals New York Academy of Sciences* 794 (September 20, 1996): 291.
3. Joseph Biederman, Stephen Faraone, Sharon Milberger, Jennifer Garcia Jelton, Lisa Chen, Erick Mick, Ross Greene, and Donald Russell, "Is Childhood Oppositional-Defiant Disorder a Precursor to Adolescent Conduct Disorder? Findings from a Four-Year Follow-up Study of Children with ADHD," *American Academy of Adolescent Psychia-try* 35, no. 9 (September 1996): 1193.

Chapter 15

1. Jerry M. Weiner, editor, *Textbook of Child and Adolescent Psychiatry* (Washington, D.C.: American Psychiatric Press, 1991), 276.

2. Ibid.
3. Rolf Loeber and Dale Hay, "Key Issues in the Development of Aggression and Violence from Childhood to Early Adulthood," *Annual Review of Psychology* 48 (1997): 375–376.
4. Weiner, *Textbook,* 277.
5. Donald Greydanus, Helen Pratt, Dilip Patel, and Mark Sloane. "The Rebellious Adolescent: Evaluation and Management of Oppositional and Conduct Disorders," *Adolescent Medicine* 44, no. 6 (December 1997): 1457, 1461.
6. Weiner, *Textbook,* 276.
7. Douglas Langbehn et al., "Distinct Contributions of Conduct and Oppositional Defiant Symptoms to Adult Antisocial Behavior: Evidence from an Adoption Study," *Archives of General Psychiatry* 55 (September 1998): 828.
8. Weiner, *Textbook,* 277.

Chapter 16

1. David Kinney, "Just Trying to Fit In, Teenage Girl Became Torture, Slaying Victim," *Seattle Times,* January 18, 1999, A6.
2. Gina Barton, "14-Year-Old Too Much for State's Juvenile Justice System," *South Bend Tribune,* November 6, 1998, D1.
3. Magda Campbell, Nilda Gonzalez, and Raul Silva, "The Pharmacologic Treatment of Conduct Disorders and Rage Outbursts," *Psychiatric Clinics of North America: Pediatric Psychopharmacology* 15, no. 1 (March 1992): 69.
4. Jerry M. Weiner, editor, *Textbook of Child and Adolescent Psychiatry* (Washington, D.C.: American Psychiatric Press, 1991), 288.
5. Ibid., 280–282.
6. Ibid., 288.
7. Daniel Connor and Ronald Steingard, "A Clinical Approach to the Pharmacotherapy of Aggression in Children

and Adolescents," *Annals New York Academy of Sciences* 794 (September 20, 1996): 292.

8. Deborah Gorman-Smith, Patrick Tolan, Rolf Loeber, and David Henry, "Relation of Family Problems to Patterns of Delinquent Involvement Among Urban Youth." Journal of Abnormal Child Psychology 26, no. 5 (1998): 319–320.

9. Campbell et al. "The Pharmacologic Treatment," 69–70.

10. Alan E. Kazdin, "Practitioner Review: Psychosocial Treatments for Conduct Disorder in Children," *Journal of Child Psychology and Psychiatry* 38, no. 2 (1997): 161.

11. Elizabeth Brestan and Sheila Eyberg, "Effective Psychosocial Treatments of Conduct-Disordered Children and Adolescents: 29 Years, 82 Studies, and 5,272 Kids," *Journal of Clinical Psychology* 27, no. 2 (1998):183–185.

12. Kazdin, "Practitioner Review," 163–168.

13. Robin Karr-Morse and Meredith Wiley, *Ghosts in the Nursery: Tracing the Roots of Violence* (New York: Atlantic Monthly Press, 1997): 8.

14. "Community Connections," *Seattle Times* (27 April 1998): B3.

15. Carina Evens and Ann Vander Stoep, "Risk Factors for Juvenile Justice System Referral among Children in a Public Mental Health System," *Juvenile Justice Referral II, The Journal of Mental Health Administration* 24, no. 4 (Fall 1997): 443.

16. David Hall and Margaret Lynch, "Violence Begins at Home," *British Medical Journal* 316 (May 23, 1998): 1551.

17. Madhu Jain and Ramesh Vinayak, "Children: Growing Up in Anger," *India Today* (July 27, 1998): 66.

Chapter 17

1. Jerry M. Weiner, editor, *Textbook of Child and Adolescent Psychiatry* (Washington, D.C.: American Psychiatric Press, 1991), 304.

2. Dante Cicchetti and Vicki Carlson, *Child Maltreatment: Theory and Research on the Causes and Consequences of*

Child Abuse and Neglect (Cambridge: Cambridge University Press, 1989), 38–39.

3. Ibid., 69.

4. David Hall and Margaret Lynch, "Violence Begins at Home," *British Medical Journal* 316 (May 23, 1998): 1551.

5. David Finkelhor and Lucy Berliner, "Research on the Treatment of Sexually Abused Children: A Review and Recommendations," *Journal of the American Academy of Child and Adolescent Psychiatry* 34, no. 11 (November 1995): 1408.

6. *Adolescent Maltreatment—Youth as Victims of Abuse and Neglect* (Washington, D.C.: U.S. Department of Health and Human Services, 1997), part 1, 3.

7. Jim Loney, "Teenagers Accused of Rape Blame Jerry Springer Show," *Times Colonist* (Victoria, Canada), January 8, 1999, A11.

8. *Adolescent Maltreatment—Youth as Victims of Abuse and Neglect* (Washington, D.C.: U.S. Department of Health and Human Services, 1997), part 1 (of 11): 3.

9. Sylvia Ann Hewlett and Cornell West, *The War Against Parents: What We Can Do for America's Beleaguered Moms and Dads,* (New York: Mariner Books Company, 1998): 231–232.

10. Peggy O'Mara, "An Epidemic of Violence," *Mothering* 95 (July/August 1999): 7.

11. Robin Karr-Morse and Meredith Wiley, *Ghosts in the Nursery: Tracing the Roots of Violence.* (New York: Atlantic Monthly Press, 1997).

Chapter 18

1. Magda Campbell, Nilda Gonzalez, and Raul Silva, "The Pharmacologic Treatment of Conduct Disorders and Rage Outbursts," *Psychiatric Clinics of North America: Pediatric Psychopharmacology* 15, no. 1 (March 1992): 70;

and Alan E. Kazdin, *Conduct Disorders in Childhood and Adolescence* (London: Sage,1987), 171.

2. Daniel Connor and Ronald Steingard, "A Clinical Approach to the Pharmacotherapy of Aggression in Children and Adolescents," *Annals New York Academy of Sciences* 794 (September 20, 1996): 298.

3. Campbell et al., "The Pharmacologic Treatment," 297.

4. Adrian Raine, Patricia Brennan, Brigitte Mednick, and Sarnoff Mednick, "High Rates of Violence, Crime, Academic Problems and Behavioral Problems in Males with Both Early Neuromotor Deficits and Unstable Family Environments," *Archives of General Psychiatry* 53 (June 1996): 548.

5. Frank A. Elliott, "Violence: The Neurologic Contribution: An Overview," *Archives of Neurology* 49 (June 1992): 602.

6. Leslie Sowers, "The Mental Health of Children: The Little Ones," *Houston Chronicle,* August 10, 1998: 1.

7. Leslie Sowers, "The Mental Health of Children: The Little Ones; An Overview: Research, Advocates, and Intervention," *Houston Chronicle,* May 17, 1998: 6.

Chapter 21

1. Alan E. Kazdin, "Practitioner Review: Psychosocial Treatments for Conduct Disorder in Children," *Journal of Child Psychology and Psychiatry* 38, no. 2 (1997): 171.

2. Lewis P. Lipsitt, editor, *Violence: Its Causes and Cures. The Brown University Child and Adolescent Behavior Letter* (Providence, RI: Manisses Communications Group, 1994), 91.

3. Richard Seven, "Miracles on 23rd Avenue: A Dynamic Church Helps Transform a Troubled Crossroads in Seattle's Central Area," *Seattle Times,* January 17, 1999, 12-19.

4. Brenda Paik Sunoo, "On a Solid Foundation: A Conversation with Wayne B. Jonas, the Departing Director of NCCAM," *Alternative Healthcare Management* (January 1999): 27.

5. Peggy O'Mara, "Children Who Kill," *Mothering* (July–August 1998): 6–9.

Index

Note to reader: Homeopathic medicines appear in italics.

About the Authors

Judyth Reichenberg-Ullman, ND, DHANP, MSW, and Robert Ullman, ND, DHANP, are licensed naturopathic physicians and board-certified diplomates of the Homeopathic Academy of Naturopathic Physicians. Dr. Reichenberg-Ullman received a doctorate in naturopathic medicine from Bastyr University in 1983 and a master's in psychiatric social work from the University of Washington in 1976. Dr. Ullman received his naturopathic medical degree from the National College of Naturopathic Medicine in 1981 and completed graduate coursework in psychology at Bucknell University in 1975. Each had extensive experience in conventional mental health settings prior to becoming naturopathic physicians.

Past president and vice president of the International Foundation for Homeopathy and past faculty members of Bastyr University, they teach, write, and lecture widely. The doctors are frequent guests on radio shows across the United States. Dr. Reichenberg-Ullman was featured on National Public Radio's *Talk of the Nation* as well as a Public Broadcasting System program examining the psychiatric labeling of children. They have written over 250 articles, some of which have been featured in national health magazines, and they have been columnists for *The Townsend Letter for Doctors and Patients* since 1990, as well as for *Resonance* and *Homeopathy Today*.

Drs. Reichenberg-Ullman and Ullman are coauthors of *Prozac-Free: Homeopathic Medicine for Depression, Anxiety and Other Mental and Emotional Problems; Ritalin-Free Kids: Safe and Effective Homeopathic Medicine for ADD and Other Behavioral and Learning Problems; Homeopathic Self-Care: The Quick and Easy Guide for the Whole Family;* and *The*

Patient's Guide to Homeopathic Medicine, which is used widely by homeopathic practitioners. You can order their books through Picnic Point Press, 131 3rd Ave., N, Edmonds, WA 98020, at (800) 398-1151, if they are not on the shelf of your local bookstore.

The doctors practice at the Northwest Center for Homeopathic Medicine in Edmonds, Washington, where they specialize in homeopathic family medicine. They treat patients by telephone consultation when there is no qualified practitioner nearby. For consultations, call (425) 774-5599. Their Web site is http://www.healthy.net/jrru.

The doctors have been married for thirteen years and reside with their two lovable golden retrievers just north of Seattle in Edmonds, Washington, which overlooks beautiful Puget Sound and the Olympic Mountains.

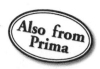
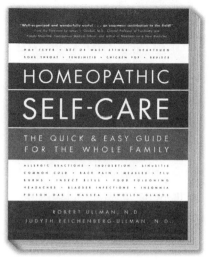

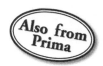
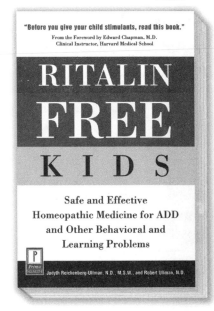

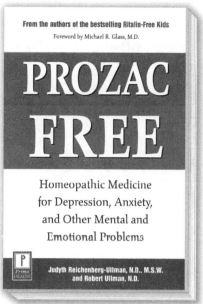

To Order Books

Please send me the following items:

Quantity	Title	Unit Price	Total
_____	**Homeopathic Self-Care**	$ **18.00**	$ _____
_____	**Ritalin-Free Kids**	$ **15.00**	$ _____
_____	**Prozac-Free**	$ **15.95**	$ _____
_____	_____	$ _____	$ _____
_____	_____	$ _____	$ _____

Subtotal	$ _____
Deduct 10% when ordering 3–5 books	$ _____
7.25% Sales Tax (CA only)	$ _____
8.25% Sales Tax (TN only)	$ _____
5% Sales Tax (MD and IN only)	$ _____
7% G.S.T. Tax (Canada only)	$ _____
Shipping and Handling*	$ _____
Total Order	$ _____

*Shipping and Handling depend on Subtotal.

Subtotal	Shipping/Handling
$0.00–$29.99	$4.00
$30.00–$49.99	$6.00
$50.00–$99.99	$10.00
$100.00–$199.99	$13.50
$200.00+	Call for Quote

Foreign and all Priority Request orders:
Call Customer Service
for price quote at 916-632-4400

This chart represents the total retail price of books only
(before applicable discounts are taken).

By Telephone: With American Express, MC or Visa,
call 800-632-8676 or 916-632-4400. Mon–Fri, 8:30–4:30.

WWW: http://www.primapublishing.com

By Internet E-mail: sales@primapub.com

By Mail: Just fill out the information below and send with your remittance to:

Prima Publishing
P.O. Box 1260BK
Rocklin, CA 95677

Name _____

Address_____

City _____ State _____ ZIP_____

American Express/MC/Visa# _____ Exp. _____

Check/money order enclosed for $_____ Payable to Prima Publishing

Daytime telephone _____

Signature _____